OXFORD MEDICAL PUBLICATIONS

DATE DUE

DEC 1 7 2002	
JUL 1 3 2004	
FEB 2 6 2009	
JUN 1 6 2010	
MAY 0 9 2012	
MAR 0 6 2015	
11-12-15	

BRODART, CO. Cat. No. 23-221-003

LUPUS

the**facts**

Graham Hughes
Lupus Research Unit,
St Thomas' Hospital, London

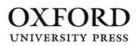

OXFORD
UNIVERSITY PRESS

OXFORD
UNIVERSITY PRESS

Great Clarendon Street, Oxford, OX2 6DP

Oxford University Press is a department of the University of Oxford.
It furthers the university's objective of excellence in research, scholarship,
and education by publishing worldwide in

Oxford New York

Athens Auckland Bangkok Bogotgí Buenos Aires Calcutta
Cape Town Chennai Dares Salaam Delhi Florence Hong Kong Istanbul
Karachi Kuala Lumpur Madrid Melbourne Mexico City Mumbai
Nairobi Paris Saõ Paulo Singapore Taipei Tokyo Toronto Warsaw

and associated companies in Berlin Ibadan

Published in the United States
by Oxford University Press Inc., New York

A catalogue record for this book is available from the British Library

Library of Congress Cataloging in Publication Data
Hughes, Graham R. V. (Graham Robert Vivian)
Lupus / Graham Hughes.
p.   cm. — (The facts)
Includes bibliographical references.
1. Systemic lupus erythematosus Popular works.   I. Title.
II. Series: Facts (Oxford, England)
RC924.5.L85H84   1999   616.7′7—dc21   99–39046

ISBN 0 19 263145 4 (Pbk)

Typeset by EXPO Holdings, Malaysia
Printed in Great Britain
on acid-free paper by
Biddles Ltd. Guildford & King's Lynn

Acknowledgements

This book is dedicated to my wife, Monica. It is dedicated to my clinical and research team and to Sandra Hampson, my secretary, who not only prepared the manuscript but advised on all aspects of the book.

It is dedicated to Julia Schofield whose advice and inspiration has opened up new dimensions (at least for me) in modern communications, together with her team, especially Justin Flute.

It is dedicated to Sally Neubert and all those who have worked to raise funds for our research charity (the St Thomas' Lupus Trust). It is dedicated to Cheryl Marcus and the many like her who organize and run patients' societies throughout the world. Above all, it is dedicated to lupus patients.

the**facts**

CONTENTS

Contents

Part I
Introducing Lupus

1
Ten common questions

Introduction

Many patients, when first told they have lupus or systemic lupus erythematosus (SLE) not unnaturally make for one or other of the standard textbooks in the public library and read a catalogue of doom and disaster: or worse, the book may contain little useful information at all. Until recent years, lupus was widely regarded, by doctors and patients alike, as a rare 'small-print' disease. Sadly, some doctors still regard it as a dire disease, relentlessly progressing to involve the kidneys, and usually fatal. Their patients are, of course, advised against pregnancy, at all costs, and given other alarming warnings.

So wrong is this overall impression that one sometimes wonders whether we are now dealing with the same disease. Indeed, in the majority of patients, the disease has a relatively benign course and a normal life expectancy.

What has brought about this change?

During the past twenty-five years, more sensitive blood tests have allowed us to recognize that, for every patient with severe or 'florid' lupus, there are many, many more with subtle forms of the disease. Indeed, it is not unreasonable to estimate that the majority of lupus sufferers are probably going about their daily routine undiagnosed.

1. What is lupus?

Lupus is a disease in which the immune system becomes over-active. It can cause clinically obvious problems, such as skin rashes, hair loss, joint swellings, chest pain, and fever, as well as more difficult to diagnose features like tiredness, depression, and muscle aches. It can also affect delicate organs such as the kidney, and its previous 'bad' reputation is based heavily on the fact that, until as recently as thirty years ago, lupus was often not diagnosed until the patient had already developed advanced kidney disease. To find out about the symptoms and effects of lupus see Chapter 2.

2. Who suffers from lupus?

People of any age can suffer from the disease. However, women out-number men by nine to one. It is a disease of childbearing age (15–40) years, and it is especially common for the disease to appear for the first time in the early twenties. This large female-to-male ratio seems to be the same in every country in the world. Chapters 11, 12, and 13 give further information about lupus in children, men, and older people.

3. What is the cause?

The cause is not known. However, there is a faint but definite genetic tendency. There are some families, for example, in which the mother and daughter suffer from the disease. Despite years of research, no virus or infectious cause has been identified. Neither is there a single strong candidate as an environmental cause. Whatever the trigger, the basic problem is an alteration in the immune system. The normal immune system which produces anti-bodies against foreign invaders, such as bacteria, goes into 'over-drive' and produces too many antibodies. Lupus has often been described as the opposite of AIDS. This is a rather daunting and inappropriate description, partly because the two diseases have so little in common, and, secondly, because the majority of lupus patients have a normal lifespan.

4. Is there a cure?

No—but this is not to say that the disease cannot be brought under control. Often lupus smoulders like embers for several years but, if the disease is treated adequately during this critical period, symptoms settle and drugs can be withdrawn. Many lupus patients in their forties and fifties come off all therapy. In Chapters 5 and 6 treatment of lupus is covered and in Chapter 21 some of the new ideas being researched are discussed.

5. How Is lupus diagnosed and monitored?

Once the possible diagnosis of lupus is considered, blood tests are used both for confirmation as well as for monitoring of the progress of the illness.

The standard screening test, the ANA (antinuclear antibody) test only takes a drop of blood, is performed in every major hospital in the world, and is cheap. If a positive test is found, other, more specific blood tests are carried out to pinpoint more accurately the extent and type of disease (see Chapter 3).

6. How is lupus treated?

The treatment of lupus aims to suppress the overactive immune system and diminish any inflammation. In the early stages lupus usually needs medical treatment. Often this treatment is 'aggressive' (e.g. the use of steroids), but later on milder drugs are used, such as antimalarials (a surprisingly useful group of medicines in lupus) and, in many patients, the treatment is ultimately discontinued. Time and time again, in the short space of this book, mention will be made of the fluctuating course of lupus. In many ways the biggest 'advance' in the treatment has been the recognition that most patients do get better and that long-term, aggressive treatment may not be required. Details about treatment are given in Chapters 5 and 6.

7. Does diet affect lupus?

Yes—although diet is often a contentious issue, with doctors, on the one hand, being somewhat suspicious of dietary cures and, on the other, the media being avid in their pursuit—there is no doubt that, in lupus in particular, diet plays a part. It is clear that lupus patients are particularly allergy-prone. Amongst allergic reactions, two of the commonest are caused by sulphonamides and Septrin, with obvious symptoms of lupus sometimes developing within hours of ingestion. There are some patients with definite food allergies. Diet is a subject which will be dealt with again in Chapters 7 and 8.

8. Can I have children?

For most patients the answer is yes. This is a far cry from the old views still current in many textbooks. At St Thomas' Hospital, as in some other teaching hospitals, there is a weekly lupus pregnancy clinic and there is something of an 'epidemic' of pregnancies in these lupus patients. More of this in Chapters 9 and 10.

9. Will my children develop lupus?

For most people, the answer is no. Lupus does not have a strong 'genetic tendency' seen in many other diseases. Nevertheless, there are some families, in whom more than one member has lupus, and it is these families which are providing important data in research. See Chapter 10.

10. How can I help myself?

One of the major advances in the last twenty-five years has been the development of lupus self-help groups throughout the world. Every continent now has these groups and, even for those who wish to keep their illness to themselves, help can be obtained in terms of leaflets, booklets, and information guides. Many countries provide a network of patient helpers who can provide that all-important direct contact at a 'patient' level, rather than having to speak to doctors, nurses, or other clinical professionals. There are many other ways of self-help, such as the avoidance of excess sunlight. We know that stress often makes lupus worse but this is far more difficult to avoid. Useful addresses are given on p. 116, providing more international contacts.

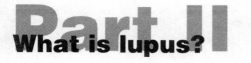

Part II
What is lupus?

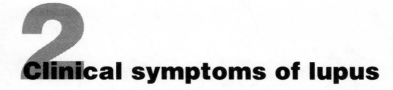

2
Clinical symptoms of lupus

General features

Although lupus is a complicated illness, capable of affecting almost every part of the body, the majority of patients suffer from a small number of the long list of features described in this book.

Lupus is a disease which can lie low for many years and then suddenly appear. Even after it has appeared, it can wax and wane. Many patients first presenting at, say, the age of twenty-five with a clear diagnosis, give past histories that are certainly suggestive of many years of the disease. The main symptoms that patients recall are 'growing pains' as children, recurrent sore throats and 'glandular fever', fainting attacks and a particular sensitivity of the skin with chilblains (cold sores in winter), and sensitivity to insect bites, etc.—'I was the one in the family who used to have a terrible time on holiday with bites'. Another feature, which many patients give, is a past history of headaches and migraine, sometimes going back to the early teens or even earlier. Finally, in some patients, the past history is one of recurrent miscarriages. This is an important subgroup of patients with lupus which will be discussed in Chapter 9.

Lupus: some general features

- Fatigue
- Skin rashes
- Hair loss
- Joint aches and pains
- Dry ('scratchy') eyes

- Inflammation of tissues covering internal organs
- Depression
- Kidney problems (e.g. swollen ankles)

Recent history

The most common presentation of lupus is of, say, a woman in her early twenties who has been on holiday in the sun and returns feeling unwell with joint pains, tiredness, muscle aches, skin rashes, and a feeling of general lethargy and depression, while acute problems are of chest pain, including pleurisy, and ankle swelling.

Malaise

Tiredness is the commonest feature of lupus. It is a major feature both early in the disease, as well as late on, and often defies explanation. There are many obvious causes, such as anaemia, joint pains, and inflammation. There may be more subtle causes such as depression. However, in some patients even the blood tests do not give a hint of abnormalities, and it is in this group of patients that diagnosis is often delayed. Indeed, many such patients are handed on from doctor to doctor and labour under a variety of diagnoses such as 'ME' (myalgic encephalitis), glandular fever, etc.

Skin rashes

These are the 'hallmark' of lupus but are not present in all patients. They can follow any pattern. The most common sites are on the palms, elbows and face. Often, the rashes are subtle (e.g. a faint pinkness may appear around the cheeks and tips of the fingers or soles of the feet.

Hair loss

One of the important diagnostic pointers to lupus is hair loss. Everybody loses hair all the time, especially when they are 'under the weather' or when there is an acute illness present. However, in active lupus, hair loss is a particular problem, not just with hair appearing in the comb, but with hair on the pillow in the morning and, even worse in some patients, with the beginning of patches of baldness. The good news is that, in the vast majority of patients, this hair loss is not permanent.

Joint pains

These vary from mild muscle aches to severe arthritis. For this reason, it is the rheumatologist who is most likely to see the patient first in a hospital setting. As we will discuss later, joint inflammation rarely leads to the damage seen in rheumatoid arthritis, for example, where permanent damage to the joint surface occurs. Take an X-ray of a lupus patient's joints and you see normal bone structure. Yet in some patients with acute lupus, the aches and pains are so severe that the patient can hardly move—'pain all over'. In this situation, it is probable that there is a combination of muscle, tendon, and joint inflammation all contributing to an almost impossible diagnostic problem. Many patients who have had severe influenza compare lupus to this acute virus disease.

'Scratchy' eyes

In many lupus patients the tear secretion is impaired. Although patients think that they cry normally, and even complain of crying more than normal, their tear secretion is nevertheless often inadequate and this leaves them with poor protection from dirt and pollution. A severe form of this dryness is called Sjögren's syndrome and is discussed in Chapter 17.

Lungs and heart

Lupus often affects the lining of the lungs (the pleura) and the heart (the pericardium). The diseases which are caused by the inflammation are often referred to as pleurisy and pericarditis. Although they are not life-threatening, they are very painful and a cause of considerable disability. Pleurisy causes sharp pain on deep breathing and this is often a feature of lupus patients. This can be a difficult diagnostic problem for doctors, as X-rays and other tests may be entirely normal. It is an important feature of the disease and often a sign of lupus activity.

Depression

This is a feature of any illness, especially a recurring or chronic one. However, over the last twenty-five years or so, it has been recognized that lupus can cause cerebral problems, usually totally reversible. These include depression.

It is an interesting fact that a number of patients with lupus, prior to diagnosis, give a history of depression which only responds once the treatment for lupus has begun. This is an important aspect of the disease and one that is often not recognized by doctors and nurses.

Ankle swelling

This can result from a number of disease processes. First, and most importantly, it may signify kidney disease. It may also be a feature of heart disease, including pericarditis, or a feature of thrombosis in the veins. Ankle swelling in lupus patients can also occur when there is joint pain involving the ankles. Mild ankle swelling is not too serious, but any doctor who sees a patient with lupus and ankle swelling needs to ensure that the kidney is not affected and a simple urine test for protein can help exclude this possibility.

Change in periods

Many young women with lupus find that their periods are altered. There may be extra (intermenstrual) bleeding or, conversely, an absence of periods for several months or even a few years. This is a common feature of lupus and gives rise to a lot of anxiety. Fortunately, in the majority of women, the periods return to normal once the disease comes under control. As with many illnesses, it appears that general disease activity seems to alter hormone balance.

Pregnancy

Because lupus affects women, often the first time that the disease becomes diagnosed is during or after pregnancy. In some women, especially those with antiphospholipid antibodies ('sticky' blood) (see Chapter 15), there is a risk of early miscarriage and the disease is sometimes first diagnosed after a woman, previously totally healthy, has suffered a number of unexplained miscarriages. Fortunately for the majority of patients, pregnancy itself provides little in the way of problems. Immediately after delivery and in the early weeks (the puerperium), there is, however, an increased risk of lupus flaring. This is the time when lupus itself can first become clinically apparent, and when doctors treating the disease need to be especially vigilant. One of the advantages of knowing the diagnosis of lupus is that these patients can be monitored closely and, if necessary, treated. Chapter 9 gives more information on pregnancy and lupus.

Lupus: some special features

- Skin (rashes, photosensitivity)
- Joints (stiffness)
- Eyes (Sjögren's syndrome)
- Blood (APS syndrome)

- Heart and lungs (pericarditis, pleurisy, artery disease)
- Kidney (inflammation, raised blood pressure)
- Brain (headache, seizures, thought disorders)

Specific features

Skin

Throughout the world, the butterfly has become the emblem of lupus groups and societies. The reason is that, in some patients, a characteristic reddish rash appears over the cheeks and nose, often strikingly in the shape of a butterfly. As with all 'classical' features of the disease, this rash by no means appears in all patients, in fact, probably the minority of lupus patients develop butterfly rashes.

The rash varies from a mild pinkness, often brought out by ultraviolet (UV) light, to a florid lumpy and disfiguring rash which comes and goes. It is a feature of active disease and usually disappears as the disease goes into remission. Rashes may affect any part of the body but other frequent sites are the V-neck area, the palms of the hands, under the elbows, and the soles of the feet. On the elbows, the rash often appears as small blisters or vesicles which come and go. Another characteristic site of these small blister-like lesions is around the tips of the fingers. Sometimes, patients give histories of chilblains, going back to their teens or even childhood. These small blistering lesions are associated with inflammation in tiny blood vessels.

The scalp may be involved and one of the characteristic features of lupus is hair loss. In addition to these rashes, there are three other distinct rashes associated with lupus:

1. *Discoid lupus* (see Chapter 16).

2. *Subacute cutaneous lupus erythematous* (SCLE). This rather cumbersome title applies to a rash, often circular and distributed on the chest, neck, and upper arms. This rash is sometimes seen in patients whose blood tests are negative. It is very sensitive to UV light. On the plus side, it is usually very responsive to antimalarials.

3. *Livedo reticularis*. This is a blotchy rash often appearing on the back of the wrists and knees. Clinically, it is found more frequently in patients with blood-clotting problems (see antiphospholipid syndrome, Chapter 15).

The skin is one of the commonest organs involved in lupus. Indeed, it has been recognized that even in those patients without obvious skin rashes, there may be very subtle skin involvement. In recent years skin biopsy (the taking of a tiny sample for laboratory testing), once a regular diagnostic procedure, has become less popular thanks to the increasing use of blood tests in lupus. It is a fact that many lupus patients have extremely sensitive skins, their history of skin sensitivity going back to childhood. Lupus patients often suffer terribly with mosquito and other insect bites, the lumps frequently lasting for days. It has often been suggested that black skin forms more sun protection and it is perhaps, at first sight, surprising, therefore, that lupus is, apparently, just as common in black as it is in white populations.

Joints

Aches and pains are the hallmark of lupus. For the vast majority of patients joint disease does not progress to endanger mobility in the same way as it often does in rheumatoid arthritis. More specifically, the inflammation within the joint does not 'burn' the cartilage or 'erode' it in the same way as it can in rheumatoid arthritis. Nevertheless, the joint pains of lupus, during the acute phase are often dramatic and in a very acute flare of lupus the patient is so severely incapacitated that he or she is immobilized until treatment is started.

Milder or 'low-grade' joint inflammation is far more common in lupus. The tendons are frequently affected, with the fingers slightly flexed. It is difficult, for example, for the patient to 'say her prayers' and flatten the fingers together. A strong indication of tendon contracture is in the thumb, and the 'hitch-hiking' thumb is a characteristic feature of lupus in some patients. Interestingly some years ago when families of lupus patients were investigated, a number of healthy family members had the same hitch-hiking thumb! Muscle aches are prominent, but the muscles themselves are rarely weakened in the way that they are in other muscle diseases, such as dermatomyositis (see Chapter 18).

Occasionally, as well as the small tendons in the hands and wrists, larger tendons, such as the Achilles (a tendon at the back of the calf and ankle) may be involved. Sometimes the patient may feel that there is difficulty in raising the toes because of the contraction of the Achilles tendon.

Eyes

Dryness of the eyes is very common. In its severest form, this is associated with a syndrome known as Sjögren's syndrome (see Chapter 17). Often the patients do not know that the tear secretion is inadequate and it requires testing with a small strip of blotting paper by the doctor to show that this is the case. It usually has no major consequences for the patient, although some people do complain of irritability of the eyes, especially in polluted environments. Some patients develop a dislike for bright lights. Examination of the eyes is extremely important in lupus patients. For example, it is the one place in the body where the blood vessels can be seen directly and any pathological abnormalities of these blood vessels can be assessed clinically by looking into the eye with an ophthalmoscope.

Blood vessels

These include arteries and veins. Inflammation of small blood vessels is common in lupus and one of the central features of the disease. In medical terms, this is given the name 'vasculitis'. The most common blood vessels to become clearly and obviously inflamed are those in the finger-tips and around the elbows. Occasionally larger, internal vessels may be involved. Another place where inflammation of blood vessels is sometimes seen is in the white of the eye, the sclera, where a red, painful inflammation can be seen, known as 'scleritis'.

A different problem, but still affecting blood vessels, is that of increased blood clotting. In some lupus patients, the blood becomes 'sticky'. The increased stickiness is easily treated if recognized (see antiphospholipid syndrome, Chapter 15).

Heart and lungs

The lining of the heart, the pericardium, is often inflamed during active flares of the disease. This shiny membrane which surrounds the heart is identical to that surrounding the lungs—the pleura—and the symptoms of 'pleurisy' and 'pericarditis' are very similar. They are characterized by sharp chest pains, often severe when the patient takes a deep breath in. Clearly, for the patient this is a very frightening symptom. It generally responds quickly to steroid treatment. It is totally different from the major 'Western disease'—coronary thrombosis or heart attack. In some patients, pleurisy may well be the first sign of a lupus flare. Again, this is one of the features of lupus which responds well to treatment, usually, in the first instance with steroids.

Are true 'heart attacks' a feature of lupus? The answer is possibly yes, in that lupus population studies have suggested a higher incidence of artery disease (including coronary artery disease) in patients in their fifties. The reasons for this increased risk are not clear, but probably include a number of factors, including prolonged steroid treatment, kidney disease and raised blood pressure in some, and 'sticky' blood (Hughes' syndrome) in others. Finally, in a group of patients with antiphospholipid antibodies, blood clots on and around the heart valves can lead to 'leaky' heart valves.

Chest infections are more common in lupus patients, especially in those receiving high doses of steroids or immunosuppressive drugs (medications used to 'dampen down' the overactive immune system). The clue to a chest infection is the development of a cough with sputum, the sputum being yellowish or green. A more serious lung manifestation of lupus is the development of a clot in the lung—characterized by acute chest pain with the production of bloody sputum. This complication of lupus is rare, and, if diagnosed correctly, quickly treated with anticoagulant drugs.

Kidney

This is the 'silent' organ in lupus. Almost all the other manifestations of lupus are recognized by patient and doctor alike. However, the inflamed kidney often produces no symptoms whatsoever. Indeed, it is an adage that pain around the kidneys is not due to the disease itself but more often suggestive of a totally different diagnosis such as a urinary tract infection or a kidney stone. Kidney inflammation in lupus is of major importance, and one of the advances during the last decade is the recognition that early, fairly aggressive treatment, especially with immunosuppressive drugs (see Chapter 5), effectively stamps out inflammation in this organ. It can be likened to smouldering embers—if treatment in the early stage is not adequate, then permanent damage occurs.

The kidney itself is only able to react to injury in a limited number of ways. First, the most common and early sign of kidney inflammation is a leaking of protein into the urine. The kidney is a complicated sieve and normally it retains protein in the blood and does not allow it to leak through into the urine. Thus, routine urine testing for protein is vital in all lupus clinics. Generally, it is good idea for patients to test their own urine with dipsticks for albumin, and this at least gives the patient the peace of mind that there is no silent kidney disease going on.

Second, another way in which the kidney reacts when inflamed is to pour out red cells, white cells, and often collections of cells (known as 'casts') into the urine. These are seen on careful microscopic examination of the urine—a vital part of any investigation of a lupus patient. If an 'active sediment' is seen (i.e. lots of cells and casts), then this is almost certainly an indication of active kidney inflammation. At this stage, the doctor may well consider a needle biopsy to be able to examine microscopically a small sample of the kidney itself in order to judge the degree of inflammation.

Third, a less subtle way in which the kidney reacts to inflammation is by causing raised blood pressure (hypertension). Blood pressure is intricately controlled and affected by the kidney. If the kidney is 'angry', blood pressure frequently rises. This, in turn, poses a further strain on the kidney and a vicious circle is in danger of setting in. For this reason, blood pressure control is one of the most vital features of the management of lupus.

One of the major reasons for the bad reputation of lupus in the past is the kidney involvement in these patients and it is understandable that, in a poor country or society, the patient may first come to the doctor in end-stage kidney failure. The decrease in severe kidney disease has been one of the major advances stemming from education of patients and doctors alike. Most textbooks say that kidney involvement occurs in about 50% of lupus patients; in my opinion, this figure is far too high. With the diagnosis of milder cases of lupus, more and more patients are being seen who have not, and will not, develop kidney disease at any time.

Brain

Inflammation in the brain provides one of the most difficult aspects of diagnosis and management of lupus. As with other organs, the small blood vessels in the brain may become inflamed and it is now thought that, in addition, some of the antibodies circulating in lupus may in some way affect brain function. Furthermore, in patients with the antiphospholipid syndrome (the clotting syndrome, see Chapter 15), there is a danger of thrombosis of the small blood vessels of the brain, in this instance leading to the possibility of permanent damage.

Like the kidney, the brain only has certain ways of objecting to disease attack. The patient can develop headaches, movement disorders, seizures (fits), depression or thought disorders, varying from the severe (psychosis) to the most subtle, cognitive disorders.

Headaches are a major feature of lupus and often precede the diagnosis by many years. In some patients, these are full-blown migraines with flashing lights, nausea, and vomiting. But in many more patients, they are 'migraine-like' with the patient still incapacitated but not as severely as in a full migraine attack. It is not uncommon to see a patient who has had a history of teenage migraine going into remission for ten or twelve years and then being diagnosed as having lupus in his or her thirties. Recent research has shown that in some patients with migraine there is a disorder of the blood-clotting system involving the platelets, and new treatments are now being directed towards this aspect of the disease.

Seizures and movement disorders are, obviously, far more severe and frightening. Normally, a seizure occurs during the very acute initial phases of lupus when the disease has come up in a major flare. The seizures vary from a full-blown epileptic fit with movement disorders, unconsciousness, tongue-biting, etc., through to far more subtle disturbances, such as periods of absence (petit mal). In the vast majority of patients, the seizures stop when the lupus itself is adequately treated. Of course, a seizure presents a major problem as far as future vehicle driving is concerned. In many countries a driving licence is not allowed for several years after a seizure. Clearly, in a lupus patient, where it is unlikely that future seizures will occur, this presents a major problem. In the vast majority of patients, it can be said that when the disease comes under control, the chances of a further fit are negligible.

One of the most recently recognized features of lupus is the breadth of presentations of neuropsychiatric involvement in the disease. Many patients with lupus suffer from depression during the acute phase and this may become profound and require psychiatric treatment. There are, however, some patients in whom brain inflammation takes a different form of thought disturbances. Agoraphobia (fear of open spaces) and claustrophobia (fear of closed spaces), for example, can be very severe in some patients, and it may take many forms, such as fear of driving on a motorway, and so on. In some patients, the thought disorder may be so severe that there are hallucinations, both 'voices' and visual hallucinations, and in others, the diagnosis of schizophrenia is made. It cannot be stressed too strongly that, in these patients, the disease ultimately has a good prognosis and with adequate treatment is reversible. One of the major worries of lupus is that those patients whose first presentation is with schizophrenia or neuropsychiatric disease who are not diagnosed, end up being possibly inappropriately treated in long-term mental hospitals. In my view, this is one of the major, future lines of research in lupus, which may not only help lupus patients, but throw light on some of the other much more widespread neuropsychiatric disorders.

Other organs

The lymph glands and spleen may be enlarged, especially in the acute phase of lupus, and often the first diagnosis made is one of glandular fever. Surprisingly perhaps, the liver is rarely affected in lupus. Thus, if a doctor finds jaundice or abnormal liver tests in a patient, alternative diagnoses such as a virus infection, etc. must be considered. All components of the blood may be affected in lupus with lowering of the white cell, platelet, and red cell counts. These are discussed in more detail in Chapter 3

Part III

How is lupus diagnosed?

3
Diagnostic tests in lupus

Introduction

The standard diagnostic tests for lupus are the so-called 'antinuclear antibodies' (ANA). These are discussed separately in Chapter 4. This chapter concentrates on the other general blood and laboratory tests which a lupus patient may be asked to undertake.

Tests for lupus

- Erythrocyte sedimentation rate (ESR)
- C-reactive protein (CRP)
- Red and white blood cell count
- Platelet count
- Urine
- Complement
- MRI scan

Erythrocyte sedimentation rate (ESR)

This test is not specific for lupus. A raised ESR or 'sed' rate may be seen in anything from influenza to malaria to rheumatoid arthritis, but in the context of a known diagnosis of lupus, it serves as a useful monitor. The ESR is the blood test most commonly used to separate inflammation from non-inflammation. If there is inflammation present (whether it be influenza, malaria, lupus or appendicitis, for example) the red cells sediment in the blood at a higher rate. This very simple test involves putting the blood in a tall tube and letting it stand. If the patient is unwell the red cells sediment more quickly.

The standard measurement is therefore called the erythrocyte (red cell) sedimentation rate or ESR. In a healthy person the rate is 20 mm per hour or less. When there is a lot of inflammation, such as in severe arthritis, that figure can rise to 120 mm or thereabouts. This is a very simple, though crude test and it does have some limitations. For example, there are some patients who are very ill but have a normal ESR, and conversely, others in whom there is no obvious clinical problem where the ESR is constantly raised, even as high as 70–80 mm per hour. Having said this, the test is a useful, general guide in the clinic and one which gives an early indication that something is wrong.

C-reactive protein (CRP)

Another sign of inflammation is the rise of a number of proteins in the blood. This seems to be secondary to a 'message' from the liver which, for undetermined reasons, provides an increased amount of these so-called 'acute phase' proteins. One of the proteins is called C-reactive protein (CRP) and has been known about for many years. Like the ESR, the CRP level goes up in acute inflammation. Oddly, in lupus the level does not generally rise unless there is infection present. This provides a useful diagnostic test. For instance, in a sick patient coming into our hospital as an emergency, a high ESR may be indicative of a whole variety of diseases. If, however, the CRP remains low it suggests lupus as the main diagnosis. If it is high, then this is a strong indication that infection may also be present.

Red cells and haemoglobin

A low haemoglobin (the red pigment in the blood) level is a marker for anaemia. In lupus, the haemoglobin level may fall and there are a number of reasons for this. First, in any illness, especially a chronic illness, the haemoglobin tends to fall. A second possibility, and much more acute, is that the haemoglobin may fall due to bleeding. Unfortunately, the most common cause of this today is from drugs, especially the non-steroidals and aspirin which can and do cause stomach bleeding. A third, though rarer cause in lupus, is the so-called 'haemolytic anaemia', where antibodies attack the red blood cells themselves. This form of anaemia can be very acute and requires aggressive treatment to reduce and remove the offending antibodies.

It is obvious that not all forms of anaemia are due to bleeding or iron deficiency and it needs careful blood testing to disentangle the various causes. Although many patients routinely take iron and vitamin supplements, it is true that in a number of patients the iron is not necessary, and medical advice is required regarding the appropriate treatment of anaemia.

White blood cells

The normal white blood count level varies widely between about 4000 and 11 000 per cc, but patients with active lupus often have a low white cell count. Indeed, it is common in a lupus clinic to see patients with a white cell count of between 1000 and 3000. The job of the white cells is protection against bacteria, foreign antigens, etc. Thus, a very low white cell count may well be associated with an increased tendency to infection. Just to make things more difficult for doctors managing lupus patients, some of the drugs used, such as azathioprine and cyclophosphamide (see Chapter 5) can themselves reduce the white cell count. Obviously, this demands very careful monitoring—walking a tightrope between the effects of the drugs and the severity of the lupus. Infection and high doses of steroids, conversely, can increase the white blood count and a lupus patient with a white cell count of 12 000 to 15 000 may well be harbouring an infection.

Platelets

Platelets are the microscopic twig-like particles in the bloodstream which are vital for the formation of a blood clot. In any blood clot, the platelets, by sticking together to form a mesh, form the basis or 'skeleton' of the clot. The normal platelet count is 150 000 or thereabouts. In some patients the platelet count often falls slightly (e.g. to between 90 000 and 100 000). In other cases, the count plummets catastrophically down to 7000 or 10 000; this condition is called 'thrombocytopenia'. Very low platelet counts may well make the patient prone to bleeding. Small blood vessels in the skin may bleed giving a small red, spotty rash (purpura). In some patients, purpura is the very first sign of lupus and these patients may be treated for a number of years under the diagnosis of 'idiopathic thrombocytopenic purpura' (ITP), the word 'idiopathic' meaning that the cause of the purpura is not known. Some of these patients may well develop lupus in later years, and patients with ITP are usually monitored continually by haematologists with regular testing for lupus. The low platelet count in lupus is usually first treated by steroids and, fortunately, responds quickly in the majority of cases.

Urine testing

Urine testing is absolutely vital in lupus patients. It is advisable that most patients should learn how to do their own dipstick testing of urine. Dipsticks are small, litmus-like paper strips that can be dipped into a sample of urine and, on changing colour, show whether there is protein or not in the urine. The earliest signs of lupus affecting the kidney are usually seen in the urine with a 'leaking' of protein.

More acute or serious inflammation in the kidney results in the appearance of red and white cells in the urine and, for this reason, a sample is sent off to the laboratory for microscopic analysis. Sometimes, these red and white cells stick together in the kidney tubules and are passed out as little collections of cells or 'casts'. These casts are a very important and significant indicator of kidney inflammation. In most lupus practices, the persistent appearance of casts is an indication for a kidney biopsy where this has not been previously done. Where there is a high level of protein in the urine, it is advisable to go on to a more precise protein measurement in a 24-hour urine sample. This cumbersome test involves the patient passing urine during a 24-period into a container, which is then taken off to the laboratory to measure the number of grams per day of protein being passed.

Complement

'Complement' are a series of proteins believed to play a part in immune defences.

In active lupus, the levels of some of these proteins fall (the two commonly measured proteins are C3 and C4). The reason for the low levels in lupus are complex and unclear, but in clinical practice, a rapidly falling C3 or C4 level often provides a clear warning signal of an impending or actual flare of the disease.

Other blood tests

Nowadays, most clinics find it cheaper and more convenient to do a routine blood screen. This includes a variety of blood tests, including calcium, cholesterol, liver function tests, kidney function tests, full blood count, ESR, uric acid, and several others. Any or all of these may become abnormal for a variety of reasons. For example, uric acid can be very high if there is impairment of the kidney function. The calcium can be low if the blood albumin is low, and so on. In other words, each of these blood tests, if abnormal, needs explanation— usually clinically obvious to the physician, but sometimes requiring some detective work.

MRI scans

Magnetic resonance imaging (MRI) (the 'scanner' as it is known to most people) has been a revolution in medicine. It has allowed exquisitely clear, anatomical pictures to be obtained of almost any part of the body. In lupus, its main use, at present, is for brain imaging, where it is important to know whether there are structural problems, such as blood clots, in a lupus patient suffering from severe headaches or other 'neurological' problems. In addition to the superb definition in the pictures obtained, the technique has the attraction of not using X-ray radiation.

4
Antinuclear antibodies (ANA) explained

Introduction

The main blood tests for lupus are the measurement of antibodies, specifically those directed against various components of the nucleus, the so-called 'antinuclear antibodies' (ANA).

The nucleus of living cells contains many chemicals, including the well-known DNA and RNA. For reasons that are still undetermined, patients with lupus produce antibodies which are directed against a number of these molecules. Antibodies against DNA are, very specifically, associated with the disease lupus, being only rarely found in other illnesses. Perhaps surprisingly, there is little to suggest that these antibodies damage or alter the cell's DNA, or, indeed, the function of the cells. From the clinical viewpoint however, antinuclear antibodies, particularly anti-DNA antibodies, are diagnostically extremely important in lupus.

Historically, the first blood investigation for lupus was the LE test (lupus erythematosus test), discovered by doctors in the United States Mayo Clinic in 1948. This was an examination of the blood, under a microscope, which showed a peculiar white cell. Essentially, this rather cumbersome and expensive test (requiring much technician time, and not totally specific) was the result of the action of circulating ANA on the cell nucleus. This test was overtaken a number of years ago by more sensitive, and certainly far cheaper ANA tests. The measurement of an ANA is the 'screening' test for lupus. If it is positive the physician must pursue more specific tests to define the disease more precisely.

Antinuclear antibody test (ANA test)

At this most simple, this very inexpensive test involves the taking of a drop of blood serum from the patient suspected of having lupus, putting it on a slide with a sample tissue present. So as to cut down on expense, there are mass-production slides available with tissue samples on them ready for laboratories to use. After leaving the serum to react with the cell nuclei on the slides, a 'marker' chemical is then added which fluoresces under ultraviolet (UV) light if there is anti-body sticking to the nucleus, and which can be 'read' by a technician looking down a microscope, or nowadays by machine.

This test is very sensitive and it is only a minority of patients with active lupus who have negative antinuclear antibody test results. Throughout the world, ANA has become the screening test for lupus and patients with active lupus generally (though not invariably) have high levels of antinuclear antibodies. Unfortunately, the ANA test, although a very useful screening device, is not specific to lupus. By far the commonest causes of positive ANA, other than lupus, are other connective tissue diseases, especially Sjögren's syndrome (a milder lupus-like disease—see Chapter 17). This probably accounts for many of the positive ANA tests seen in patients over the age of forty. Other rheumatic diseases, notably rheumatoid arthritis, may also give positive antinuclear antibodies and, in some diseases, the percentage of positives is high. The finding of a positive ANA, therefore, must lead the physician to pursue more specific antibody tests, such as the DNA antibody and ENA (extractable nuclear antigens) tests.

DNA antibodies

DNA

The 'double helix' is the most important chemical in the nucleus of the cell, being the scaffolding on which the genetic code is built up—a code which is then handed on from parent to offspring. It is one of the interesting findings of nature that lupus patients develop anti-bodies directed against DNA. This finding has resulted in major advances, not only in the diagnosis of lupus but in the understanding of some aspects of molecular biology. It was in the late 1960s that a number of research workers found that lupus sera were able to react with double-stranded (double-helix) DNA. Other diseases that cause diagnostic confusion with SLE, such as rheumatoid arthritis, did not produce these antibodies. Thus, antibodies to DNA became not only the hallmark of lupus, but one of the most disease-specific tests in the whole of medicine.

In 1969, the DNA binding test was devised. This consists of the adding of serum to radioactive DNA and thereby, with the use of a counter, measuring the amount of binding of the antibody to the DNA molecule. This gives us, in clinical practice, a figure— the DNA binding value—which provides a useful guide to the activity of lupus. In simplistic terms, blood tests can show a DNA binding value of between 0% and 100%:0% is normal and 100% indicates active lupus. Obviously, in real life, it is never quite as simple as this, but, in general terms, DNA binding values are very valuable in the individual patient for monitoring month-to-month progress. A rapidly rising titre is a red warning light. A fall to negative usually indicates the progress of the disease towards remission.

Extractable nuclear antigens (ENA)

I will never forget being floored by an old physician and a dear friend who once asked me 'is ENA the next thing after DNA?'. As usual, the development of more specific tests for the various anti-bodies directed against the various proteins and chemicals in the nucleus and cytoplasm of the cell threw up a lot of different patterns. In a series of clinical and laboratory observations, led, in particular, by two American researchers, Drs Eng Tan and Morris Reichlin in the early 1970s, it was recognized that some lupus patients showed antibodies which differed from those directed against DNA. By taking 'ground-up' nuclei (e.g. spleen extract), they were able to show that some patients with lupus and lupus-like diseases showed reactivity against a variety of cell chemicals (proteins and nucleoproteins) other than DNA, and that these patterns often coincided with important clinical features. Today, these ENA have now been well characterized and (especially anti-Ro) are of immense value to the specialist in lupus. Some of the more important subsets of these antibodies are described here.

Anti-Ro (anti-SSA)

This particular antibody is of great importance in connective tissue diseases. 'Ro' is the name given to an RNA protein which exists mainly in the cytoplasm and is therefore sometimes seen in patients whose conventional antinuclear antibody tests are negative. This has been strongly associated with Sjögren's syndrome (see Chapter 17), and with 'neonatal lupus' (see Chapter 9). In our own experience, it is also associated with three other features:

(1) photosensitivity,

(2) heightened allergy to some drugs, particularly Septrin, and

(3) occasionally, mild neurological abnormalities such as numbness.

Some patients with Ro antibodies have even been diagnosed as having a variant of multiple sclerosis.

How common is anti-Ro?

It occurs in about a quarter of all lupus patients. However, if it occurs on its own in the absence of DNA antibodies, it is more likely to be associated primarily with Sjögren's syndrome (symptoms include dryness of the eyes, nose, and mouth and enlarged salivary glands— see Chapter 17), or with the peculiarly photosensitive skin rash called 'subacute cutaneous LE'. Both of these conditions are relatively benign, although recurring, and for this reason, the presence of anti-Ro antibody is often regarded as a marker of milder lupus disease. A more serious, though rare, association of anti-Ro is congenital heart block. Although this occurs in a very small minority of offspring of Ro-positive mothers, there is no way of predicting the 1% or so of patients whose babies are at risk of this cardiac condition (see Chapter 9).

Anti-Sm

It is said that the antibody 'Sm' was named after a patient called Smith. Anti-Sm is found much more commonly in black and Chinese lupus populations. It is a specific test for lupus, but far less useful diagnostically than anti-DNA.

Anti-Jo 1

This particular antibody is not normally found in lupus but is found in a group of patients with muscle inflammation (dermatomyositis) and particularly in a group of those patients with muscle disease who also suffer from lung problems. Clearly, therefore, for the physician this is an important test in patients with muscle disease.

Other ENA

There are a host of 'small print' ENA now described, mostly variants of those mentioned above. The presence of an ENA in a patient or a relative suspected of having lupus or a lupus variant, is of clinical and diagnostic importance. In general, it means that there is a background tendency for autoimmune disease and, although the individual may be totally asymptomatic, the measurement of these antibodies is, at least in clinical research, providing useful information on the genetic background of autoimmune diseases.

Part IV
What is the treatment?

5
Drugs commonly used in lupus

Introduction

It must be hard for a person first diagnosed as having lupus to believe that he or she may, and often does, ultimately come off all treatment. One of the advances in our knowledge of lupus in the last three decades is the realization that the disease is cyclical and frequently subsides. In any discussion of medical treatment there are two aspects—drugs and 'non-pharmacological' treatments. This chapter will deal with the drugs which are commonly used for the actual treatment of lupus. In the next chapter a mixture of other drugs which may be used in the disease will be discussed, for example, those used to treat some of the complications of lupus such as epilepsy or blood pressure.

The medication commonly used in lupus will be considered here under four main headings:

(1) non-steroidals,

(2) antimalarials,

(3) steroids, and

(4) immunosuppressives.

In reading about medication, there will often appear to be two names for the same drug. This is because a drug will be given a trade name, (e.g. Plaquenil) and also a chemical name, in this case, hydroxychloroquine. Patients are often confused by seeing one or other name on their prescription. Trade names also often vary between countries. As a tip, a trade name will always be capitalized but not the chemical name.

> **Drugs used in the treatment of lupus**
>
> - NSAIDs (e.g. Feldene, Naprosyn, Voltarol)
> - Antimalarials (e.g. Plaquenil, Nivaquine, Atabrine)
> - Steroids (e.g. prednisolone, ACTH, methylprednisolone)
> - Immunosuppressives (e.g. Imuran, Endoxana, methotrexate, cyclosporin)

Non-steroidals (NSAIDs, non-steroidal anti-inflammatory drugs)

This rather cumbersome name has been coined for the very useful group of drugs developed to combat arthritis. They include names such as Feldene, Naprosyn, Voltarol, Relifex, Oruvail, etc. Essentially, they succeeded aspirin which, until thirty years ago, was the main treatment for arthritis. Many patients find it hard to believe that the NSAIDs are less toxic than full dose aspirin. The main problem with all the NSAID family is that they have a propensity to cause indigestion and unfortunately, more especially in older patients, stomach bleeding and even ulceration.

History of NSAIDs

High doses of aspirin, such as 12 to 14 tablets a day, were, in the past, the standard treatment for rheumatoid arthritis, juvenile arthritis, and even, in some cases, lupus. This dose of aspirin, not surprisingly, had many side effects, including drowsiness, indigestion, ringing in the ears (tinnitus), but most of all, indigestion and gastric irritation. Oddly, a number of lupus patients appeared to have an abnormal liver reaction to aspirin, the liver function tests becoming abnormal on the high doses. It is an interesting historical quirk that it took some eighty years for this side effect of aspirin to be discovered, largely, because, at the turn of the century, there were no stringent drug trial programmes as there are today for newly introduced medication. The development of NSAIDs about thirty-five years ago, came as a welcome advance in the field of rheumatology. For those patients suffering from arthritis they offered a far less indigestible and far more acceptable form of pain relief in arthritis and, not surprisingly, the pharmaceutical companies made large profits with the advent of these drugs. So many of these drugs came onto the market that it was tempting to conclude that there was little to choose between them. They were 'me too' drugs. I think this is a little nihilistic. Rather oddly, and defying the laws of science, individual patients do seem to differ in their response to these drugs. For those patients with mild to moderate arthritis, it is now recommended that, if one fails then, there is still no reason against trying another ... and even another.

Pharmacology

In general terms, the non-steroidals are safe and they do not require regular blood testing. As mentioned above, however, they can cause indigestion and this is their major drawback. Usually, the patient notices this and the drug is stopped. But occasionally, and most worryingly for all concerned, some patients develop stomach ache, and the painful symptoms of heartburn, indigestion, and so on. These adverse effects have led to a media 'backlash' and, sadly, to the feeling in the minds of many patients that all these drugs are dangerous. As usual, the truth lies somewhere in between. The effect of these drugs is on inflammation, their effect being most obvious in patients with warm, swollen, painful joints.

A major advance in recent years has come with the discovery of NSAIDs which avoid stomach toxicity (so-called COX-2 inhibitors). Two drugs in this new class are already being marketed (under the trade names 'Vioxx' and 'Celebrex') in some countries.

Antimalarials

This group of drugs plays a major part in the treatment of lupus. It must be said at the outset that the reason why these drugs should work in lupus is unclear though there are many theories. One of the first descriptions of the use of antimalarials in lupus came one hundred years ago at St Thomas' Hospital, London, when a Dr Payne published detailed clinical reports of the use of antimalarials in discoid lupus (Chapter 16), pointing out that they helped combat not only skin problems but also possibly some more general symptoms such as fever and joint pains. The family of antimalarials are all rather similar but, nevertheless, have important differences as well. They are not steroids. The three most widely used antimalarials are hydroxychloroquine (Plaquenil), chloroquine (Nivaquine), and mepacrine (Atabrine). In my practice, we have moved across almost entirely to hydroxychloroquine, as I consider this to be less indigestible and as having fewer side effects than the older drug, chloroquine. Mepacrine is a useful antimalarial but is limited by the fact that, in higher doses, it causes a yellow pigmentation of the skin and, obviously, only low doses can be given.

Hydroxychloroquine

This drug, given at a dosage of one tablet (200 mg) daily, or (less often) two tablets (400 mg) daily, is useful for those patients with severe skin lupus and with joint pains. The drug takes about two to three weeks to start working effectively but in many patients there is not only a feeling of improvement in the skin and their general well-being but also less joint pains, tiredness, muscle aches, and sometimes, where there is a temperature, less fever. The effect on skin lupus is variable but can be very dramatic indeed with a total clearing of the most severe rash. Antimalarials can be given for months and even years on end and are one of the central groups of drugs used in our lupus clinic.

Combination antimalarials

Owing to the very low eye toxicity of low dose hydroxychloroquine (see below), I tend to stick to a rather conservative dosage of one tablet (200 mg) daily, though many would advocate two per day. However, in patients with severe skin disease, such as some patients with bad discoid lupus (see Chapter 16), I use a combination of anti-malarials, such as hydroxychloroquine, 200–400 mg daily, together with mepacrine, 100 mg daily on alternate days. This could be considered to be medical 'cooking', but it is a regime which I find extremely effective in many patients whose skin condition proves resistant to more conventional doses.

Side effects of antimalarials

The main and overriding worry about the use of high doses of anti-malarials is that they can affect the retina of the eye. In the past, there were undoubted cases of eye disease, and even blindness resulting from injudicious use of antimalarials. It has become clear that hydroxychloroquine (Plaquenil) is less toxic as far as the eye is concerned than chloroquine. It is also probable that the lower doses now used are safe, though it is absolutely vital that annual eye checks are carried out by a qualified ophthalmologist. In 1996, St Thomas' Hospital completed a combined five year follow-up study of our patients on hydroxychloroquine using sophisticated electroretinography and other eye tests, and found no case of even the slightest eye damage on the low doses used.

Other side effects include indigestion (usually mild), occasional tinnitus (ringing in the ears), and sometimes headaches. An extremely rare problem is a slight skin rash or a darkening of the skin and nails, though this is only normally seen in patients on higher doses.

Finally, one rare side effect which is not widely known, even by doctors, is when hydroxychloroquine is started in moderately high doses, such as two or three tablets daily, there is a very subtle effect on the eye muscles leading to focusing difficulty or to mild double vision. Obviously, this is frightening for the patient who is already worried about eye toxicity. However, this symptom subsides if the dose is reduced.

Antimalarials have always been regarded as being contraindicated in pregnancy and in general terms this is still a wise policy. However, there are now increasing numbers of patients in clinics throughout the world who have had successful pregnancies while taking hydroxychloroquine and it appears that hydroxychloroquine is in fact safe in pregnancy.

How do antimalarials work?

The list of ways in which antimalarials work appears endless. For instance, they have immunosuppressive effects, antiviral effects, etc. However, their main effect is their ability to suppress the inflammatory process. In this respect, they are rather similar to the NSAIDs. However, an important, additional effect is their ability to protect from ultraviolet (UV) light—lupus patients can be very sun-sensitive. Although this does not provide a total protection (patients obviously cannot sunbathe all day because they are taking antimalarials) it is, nevertheless, clearly important. In some sunny countries, doctors often use antimalarials during the summer in patients with mild lupus and 'rest' the patient from the drug during the winter months. There are many variations in the way that these drugs can be given. It may well be that there is an important, though as yet poorly studied, immunosuppressive effect of antimalarials. One study in Africa showed, for example, that conventional antimalarials, as used in cases of malaria, might actually have an immunosuppressive or 'damping' effect on the response to vaccination. In other words, the person's normal immune response to a vaccine is lessened. This clearly has important implications in public health as well as in the treatment of lupus. One of the useful effects of antimalarials is that in those patients with clotting problems, such as patients with the antiphospholipid (Hughes') syndrome (see Chapter 15), antimalarials have an important (though mild) anti-clotting effect. It is interesting that Sir John Charnley, who pioneered total hip replacement, originally used antimalarial drugs to combat post-operative blood clotting in his patients. Although we do not use antimalarials as our first choice in patients whose main problem is clotting, it is useful to know that in those who have both skin lupus, as well as a mild clotting problem, there may be additional benefits to be gained by the use of drugs such as hydroxychlorquine.

Incidentally, patients taking hydroxychlorquine for lupus still require other antimalarials for travel in certain countries—this drug alone does not protect against malaria.

Steroids (corticosteroids)

Steroids (e.g. prednisolone) have revolutionized the management of lupus more than any other drug. It was probably in lupus that some of the major 'miracle cures' were seen during those heady years when steroids were discovered by Hench and colleagues, studies which were rewarded with the Nobel Prize. I am sure we all remember the stories of patients, who had previously been thought to be dangerously ill, improving within hours of the start of steroids. As everybody knows, the doses used in the past were high and the side effects many. Sadly, it is the side effects—weight gain, moon face, acne, etc.—rather than their beneficial effects, which are often now regarded as the hallmark of steroids. They are still life-saving in many patients and are still vital in the management of many, if not the majority of lupus patients at some stage during their disease. However, modern management has advanced with the use of 'steroid alternatives' and in better 'fine-tuning' of steroid dosage.

Commonly used steroids

Far and away the most commonly used steroid now is prednisolone. This is easy to take, easy to monitor, and has almost totally replaced all other forms of steroids. An injectable form of steroid, ACTH (adreno-cortico-trophic-hormone), was popular in former years. Some doctors still like to use this (e.g. on a twice-weekly injection basis). ACTH is similar to prednisolone but regarded as the more 'natural' steroid—the hormone, in fact, which is secreted by the pituitary to stimulate the adrenal gland. A third form of steroid, which is used for acute situations, is so-called 'pulse' methylprednisolone. This is a 'drip' which lasts for an hour or so and is a way of giving a large dose of steroid via the vein. This is widely used in hospital practice for the patient who is acutely ill, or a patient in whom a major 'boost' to the system is required. Doses are given of between 500 mg and 1000 mg of methylprednisolone—without, perhaps surprisingly, many side effects. Having said this, the major routine steroid throughout the world is prednisolone or prednisone (do not worry if your prescription says one or the other because they are almost totally interchangeable—in the body, prednisone is converted into prednisolone).

Doses used

The dose is variable but, to give some general examples, a very unwell patient with newly diagnosed acute lupus may require 60 mg daily, ideally reducing this to towards 40–30 mg daily over the following one to two weeks. For milder cases, such as a patient in whom diagnosed lupus has flared, a dose of between 15 mg and 20 mg daily might be given for a few weeks. In the vast majority of milder lupus cases a 'maintenance' dose of between 5 mg and 10 mg daily is the most popular choice. In the past, doses of over 80 mg were widely given but this is now regarded as excessive. High doses are extremely toxic and the chances of developing side effects, especially infections, as a result of the treatment, far outweigh the advantages gained.

Reducing steroids is an art and demands cooperation between patient and doctor. The graph is steep to start with but flattens later. For instance, it may be possible to reduce the dosage fairly quickly from 60 mg through to 40 mg or 20 mg daily, but after that the reduction must be slower, and often for patients at a daily level of 10 mg or so I tend to reduce the dosage by as little as 1 mg every month. In some countries, 1 mg tablets are not available and this is unfortunate. Fine-tuning, using these tiny amounts, is extremely important in patients and has contributed to better management. Most steroid tablets now come either in a coated form or as white tablets, and many patients feel that the coated form causes less stomach irritation.

Alternate-day steroids

The fashion for using steroids on alternate days has waxed and waned. In early studies, especially in children with arthritis, it was felt that giving alternate day steroids allowed the patient's adrenal glands to work, or at least to 'wake up'. For most lupus patients this does not appear to be necessary, and the use of alternate-day steroids seems more dependent on the doctor than on any strong scientific evidence. The problems of alternate-day steroid dosage are, first, that it is more difficult to remember to take tablets every other day, and second, some patients seem to suffer more problems on the 'non-steroid' day. That at least is my feeling.

Side effects of steroids

Low doses, such as 7.5 mg a day, have very few side effects, especially in the short-term. In fact, the patient's well-being, when steroids are first started, usually far outweighs any side effects. The two common side effects of steroids are sleep disturbance and increased appetite. In some patients, the body clock is turned upside down, the person feeling wide awake at three in the morning and sleepy at three in the afternoon.

Increased appetite applies particularly to sweet foods and, of course, weight gain is the outcome if the calorie intake is not monitored.

Other more serious side effects, usually associated with high doses over longer periods are:

(1) muscle weakness,

(2) raised blood sugar level (and sometimes diabetes),

(3) softening of the bones (osteoporosis)

Immunosuppressives

This group of drugs, which have the ability to calm the immune response, play an important part in the management of some patients with lupus. There are a large number of these drugs, and considerable experience has been built up over the years of their use, notably in patients with cancer. In general, far lower doses are used in diseases such as lupus. In common practice, the two most regularly used drugs are azathioprine (Imuran) and cyclophosphamide (Endoxana, Cytoxan). Two others, used somewhat less frequently, are methotrexate and cyclosporin.

Azathioprine (Imuran)

Azathioprine is one of the most widely used drugs in the management of lupus. Although, in common with its other colleagues in this family of drugs, it can lower the white blood cell count, it still has a very acceptable safety margin and is prescribed to a variety of patients with lupus, including children and occasionally pregnant women. The drug is given in tablet form, most commonly at a dose of 2.5 mg for each kilogram of body weight. For most people this means a dose of either two tablets a day (100 mg) or three tablets a day (150 mg).

Uses of azathioprine

Azathioprine is frequently used as a 'steroid-sparing' drug. In other words, with patients with fairly active disease, especially in those with kidney disease, it is now common practice to combine two drugs rather than simply use high dose steroids. For those patients with lupus kidney disease, it is recognized that fairly aggressive treatment early on may well reverse the inflammation in the kidney and return kidney function to normal. Azathioprine is used over a lengthy period, often for a number of years. Although it can be stopped quickly, there is some evidence that, like steroids, it is best to stop the drug in stages (e.g. down to one tablet daily for a month or two and then to stop altogether). Many trials have shown that azathioprine also has a positive effect in other aspects of lupus, such as improving the results of blood tests. It is not a steroid and has none of the major side effects of steroids, such as weight gain.

Side effects

The most important side effect is depression of the bone marrow cells with a resulting fall in white blood cell count and, less commonly, a lower platelet and red cell count. Regular blood counts are therefore imperative. Much more common is the side effect of nausea and indigestion. Although azathioprine does not cause heartburn and burning stomach problems of the non-steroidals, it does, in some patients, cause considerable nausea and a feeling of loss of appetite. This can be so severe as to require stopping the treatment. In some cases, the results from liver function tests are affected. It is important to remember that the liver itself is rarely involved in lupus and therefore abnormal results of liver tests are suggestive of another cause such as a side effect of drugs or a viral infection.

Cyclophosphamide (Endoxana)

This is a far more powerful, and more toxic, drug than azathioprine. Formerly, it was used in tablet form (oral preparation) but more recently, because of far fewer side effects, it is most commonly given as a periodic injection or 'pulse'. There has been a minor revolution in the management of lupus with a change from 'oral' to 'pulses' of intravenous cyclophosphamide.

Side effects

Cyclophosphamide affects dividing cells. It is a very powerful drug and, more so than with azathioprine, it has the capacity to reduce the blood count. It can even do this dramatically and a close watch must be kept on the use of this drug. More seriously, it can affect the dividing cells of the reproductive system, such as the ovary cells and the sperm.

In addition to the effects on the blood count and on the ovary, cyclophosphamide has many other effects, some of which are potentially very serious. These include nausea and diarrhoea and, of greater importance, sometimes marked hair loss. One very specific side effect of cyclophosphamide is on the bladder and patients taking this drug by mouth occasionally suffer from bladder irritability and even a very severe form of cystitis called 'haemorrhagic cystitis'. Many of these side effects have been overcome by a change to intravenous pulse doses.

Pulse cyclophosphamide

Over the last decade, there has been a move towards the use of intermittent injections of cyclophosphamide given as an intravenous drip. The standard regime used in our practice is lower than that used in some other centres and we tend to give a weekly injection of 500 mg for three successive weeks and thereafter a monthly injection for three to six months. The advantages of the 'drip' regime are twofold: first, it results in far fewer side effects; second, there is a drug available called Mesna which almost totally blocks the irritant effect on the bladder and the troublesome cystitis. Higher doses of cyclophosphamide, presumably because these lower the immune response, have been associated with a high frequency of infections, particularly with the virus infection, herpes zoster (shingles). Using the low dose regime we have found that the incidence of herpes zoster is negligible. In most practices, pulse cyclophosphamide is used either for a bad flare of the disease or in a new patient in order to bring the disease under control.

Methotrexate

Methotrexate, the drug which has revolutionized the management of rheumatoid arthritis because of its extraordinarily powerful effects on joint inflammation, has played less of a part in the management of lupus. However, increasing use of this drug in arthritis generally has meant that a number of lupus patients have received methotrexate. So far, the data suggest that it is of value in those lupus patients in whom arthritis is a major problem. More recently, there have been reports that it may help some of the skin rashes seen in lupus.

Cyclosporin

This drug, the 'wonder drug' in transplantation, has been used in lupus, though not as widely as might have been expected from its successful use in transplantation. It has a slightly different effect on the immune response from other immunosuppressive drugs discussed in this chapter. The data in lupus so far suggest that it has some value, though its role is yet to be fully established. Unfortunately, even in low doses, it has many side effects (including 'pins and needles'), due to its irritant effect on nerves (neuropathy) and its tendency to increase blood pressure. This increase in blood pressure is a major problem in lupus patient with kidney involvement who may already have blood pressure problems.

Other agents

The search actively goes on for newer, better immunosuppressive agents, and drugs under study include mycophenalate-mofetyl and tacrolinus, and 'biologic' agents such as anti-CD40. More of these, perhaps, in future editions of this book.

6
Other treatments

Skin creams

In those patients with lupus of the skin, it is extremely tempting to treat the condition directly (i.e. by the use of various steroid creams). Certainly, steroid creams play a major part in a whole variety of skin diseases including lupus. In discoid lupus (Chapter 16), the acute involvement and itchiness of the disease may well be eased by various steroid skin creams. It is important to remember that there are a variety of strengths of steroid dosages in the different creams. A problem with the excessive use of steroid creams is that they can actually cause damage to the skin—a degree of skin thinning—and it really is wise to obtain specialist advice in their use, rather than depend solely on self-medication.

Sun protection agents

First, a reminder that the danger time for sun effects (mainly UVB) is between 11 am and 3 pm. Most sunscreens are either organic chemicals which absorb UV (ultraviolet) light, or inorganic pigments such as titanum dioxide which absorb and scatter UV light. It has always been felt that conventional sunscreens are less than perfect, particularly in the case of the lupus patient. A recent study may provide a partial explanation: a group of dermatologists have found that we tend to apply less sunscreen than is needed to achieve the manufacturer's recommended sun protection factor. The most frequently missed areas are the back and sides of the neck, the temples and the ears—the sites often affected in lupus.

Blood pressure tablets

The management of blood pressure remains extremely complicated. For both doctor and patient, it is unfortunate that in many cases, the management of blood pressure requires two or even three different pills. The worst situation is trying to explain to an already sceptical patient that yet another tablet is required. On the positive side, it can be said that in the late 1990s, almost all blood pressure problems can be controlled. However, seriously high blood pressure does demand careful monitoring.

What levels of blood pressures are important?

When blood pressure is taken, an 'upper' and 'lower' reading are recorded. For example, a 'normal' blood pressure (e.g. 120/80) would consist of two figures, a high and a low. In general, it is the lower figure, the so-called diastolic pressure that matters. For the average adult patient, a diastolic reading of 80 is fine, a reading of 90 is 'beware', and of 100 means 'may well require regular treatment'. Diastolic figures of 110 and over always demand treatment.

There are many ways of treating blood pressure, such as the use of diuretics (or water pills) to get rid of excess fluid, drugs such as beta-blockers which affect the heart directly, and drugs such as the so-called 'calcium antagonists' which affect the blood vessels. The management of a blood pressure problem is often complicated, requiring more than one drug. All blood pressure agents have side effects. Water pills (diuretics), if overused, can cause dryness, dehydration, and an alteration to the chemistry of the body. For example, some diuretics reduce potassium resulting in cramps, and others can cause drowsiness. Fortunately, some of the newer blood pressure drugs are superior as far as their side effects are concerned. For those

patients with lupus and marked kidney disease there is hardly anything more critical than the careful management of blood pressure.
Indeed, this is probably even more important in some patients than
the management of the underlying lupus itself. A continually raised
blood pressure has, itself, a negative effect on the kidney and this, in
turn, leads to even higher blood pressure. So, the vicious circle sets
in unless it is broken by adequate treatment. In many ways, the
modern treatment of blood pressure has been one of the success
stories in the improved outlook for lupus patients.

Anticonvulsants

As mentioned in earlier chapters, various forms of epilepsy are a
problem in some lupus patients, and a small number of patients
require medium-term or even long-term anticonvulsants. There are a
variety available and, as in the case of blood pressure control, often
more than one agent is required. Again, this is a complicated subject.
There are various types of epilepsy such as grand mal (fits), petit mal
(absences) and temporal lobe epilepsy (e.g. feeling of unreality, *déjà
vu*, etc.) These different forms of epilepsy require very precise treatment. An anti-epileptic drug which we commonly use in our lupus
patients is sodium valproate which fortunately has very few side
effects. A detailed discussion of the various anticonvulsants is beyond
the scope of this book.

Gammaglobulin ('pooled' intravenous globulin)

Several years ago, it was found that the injection of gammaglobulin
(i.e. the body protein that forms the basis of antibodies—the body's
immune protein defence) sometimes had a dramatic effect on improving platelet counts in patients whose platelet levels had fallen. This
very expensive form of treatment has also been shown to be helpful in
some forms of lupus, especially in those patients whose platelet counts
fall. The rationale for this treatment is rather unclear, though gammaglobulin seems to 'swamp' or 'saturate' some of the immune receptor
sites in the body. At the moment, there is no consensus to suggest that
the widespread use of gammaglobulin should be a standard treatment in
lupus.

Anti-clotting agents

In patients with antiphospholipid (Hughes') syndrome (Chapter 15), thrombosis is a major problem. In these patients, and possibly in others, various forms of blood-thinning agents—so-called 'anticoagulants'—are required. The three commonly-used are junior aspirin, warfarin (a coumarin derivative) and heparin.

Junior aspirin

One of the major advances in the understanding of lupus in the last decade has been that some patients have a tendency for the blood to become too thick or 'sticky'. It has long been known that low dose aspirin (and it is vital to remember that this really is low dose aspirin) is highly effective. Junior aspirin (75 mg daily, i.e. a quarter of a standard adult aspirin) has an important effect on the platelets of the blood, making them less 'sticky'. Trials in patients with heart attacks, strokes, etc., indicate that this may well be an important daily medicine in avoiding further blood clots. In patients who have had clots in lupus, we now use a junior aspirin as standard therapy. Interestingly, in those women who have had recurrent miscarriages due to thrombosis of the placental vessels, low dose aspirin has also been shown to be effective in helping a number of these pregnancies to be successful.

Warfarin (Comdin)

This is the standard medicine for those people who have had a major thrombosis. This acts in a different way from aspirin, affecting the actual clotting system of the blood. In patients who have had a major clot, such as leg vein thrombosis, or a lung clot, or a stroke, it is vital that anticoagulant control is good. Once started on warfarin, patients usually have few problems if monitored carefully, usually by local hospitals which run standard anticoagulant clinics. In general, the blood needs to be kept thinner by a ratio of two to three (the so-called 'prothrombin ratio' or 'international ratio'). Obviously, if the dose is too high and the blood becomes too thin then there is a danger of bleeding, especially after minor trauma. Warfarin is a very safe medicine with few side effects, other than, of course, the danger of increased bleeding. However, it is important for the patient to know that it does interact with a number of drugs and if, for example, the patient is put on a course of antibiotics this may well affect the dosage requirement of warfarin.

Heparin

Heparin, like warfarin, affects the clotting system directly. It has to be given as an injection and is usually used in acute situations such as when the patient is first admitted to hospital, in order effect rapid anticoagulant control. It is also used during surgery as its management and its level can be more precisely monitored. It is used in pregnancy in those women with clotting problems. Warfarin cannot be given in the first part of pregnancy as it has an adverse effect on fetal development, thus in these patients heparin is used for the first part of pregnancy, often reverting back to warfarin in the later stages of pregnancy. A rare side effects of long-term heparin is softening of the bone (osteoporosis) and, for this reason above all others, long-term heparin is avoided.

A number of synthetic 'low molecular weight heparins' have been produced.

Lipid lowering agents

The realization that coronary and other arterial disease may be an important development in some lupus patients has resulted in a refocusing on management of known risk factors (stopping smoking, for example). One risk factor, raised cholesterol, is now amenable to treatment not only by diet, but by drugs known as 'statins'. These important agents may come to play a greater role in future in the management of some lupus patients.

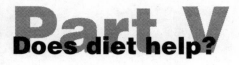
Part V
Does diet help?

7
Diet and alternative medicine

Does food affect lupus?

The answer in some cases is yes. Every patient asks whether there is a diet which helps lupus. Despite the plethora of books now available on dietary 'cures' in diseases such as rheumatoid arthritis, sadly there is no overall single, effective diet. However, there are certain obvious health warnings; those patients with a tendency to fluid retention and swelling of the legs should avoid excess salt, sometimes even to the point of reducing considerably the amount of salt in cooking. In those patients who are overweight, possibly associated with steroid use, it is imperative to try to keep the overall weight down, partly to avoid excess strain on the hip and knee joints. In patients who have had protein leaks in the urine and whose overall blood protein level is low, dietary advice is required regarding an increase of protein intake (meat, eggs, fish, etc.).

This chapter deals mainly with food allergy and possible side effects of individual foods. Lupus patients are often very 'allergic'. There is no doubt that they have a higher incidence of allergies to certain drugs, such as antibiotics, and to insect bites, pollen, etc. Often the relatives of lupus patients are themselves 'allergic'. It is perhaps not surprising therefore that there are many patients who give clear-cut histories of exacerbation of the disease following certain foods. There are no absolute rules about this, though dairy produce (especially cheese), coffee, and red wine seem to come high on the list. I always advise my patients to keep a very careful dietary record. If the disease fluctuates, for example, if there are certain days on which the joint pains or the migraines are worse, then this is possibly an indication of exacerbation caused by certain foods.

'Is there something which you have eaten over the last twenty-four hours, which might have been slightly out of the ordinary?' I have seen a number of patients, both with lupus and Sjögren's syndrome, who have genuinely managed to keep off any drugs, partly by strict observation of the foods or drinks which bring out a flare of the disease.

Some years ago, we published a case report of a patient who was crippled with rheumatoid arthritis and was on a very strong combination of medication for the arthritis. She felt that cheese possibly made her arthritis worse but was uncertain about this. She adored cheese and ate it most days! As a test, she agreed to avoid dairy produce over a period of seven weeks. To our surprise and delight, after a few weeks there was clinical improvement, and after six months she managed to reduce and finally stop all medication. Being 'good scientists' we felt that we have to prove that this was not merely coincidence and so with her permission we retested ('re-challenged') her with a number of food antigens, finally testing her with the cheese protein, 'casein'. The following day, she was rigid with severe arthritis and this lasted a few days. She is now very healthy, but if, inadvertently, there is cheese added to any food, she suffers quite marked flares of arthritis the following day. Some of the commoner symptoms of food allergy are 'irritable bowel', 'stuffy nose' or 'rhinitis', 'headaches', and 'joint pains'. These are warning signs that a patient may have a food allergy.

Unfortunately, food allergy is often complicated and the allergic patient may react to a number of food products. Throughout the world, food allergy clinics are blossoming. The main object of these clinics is to starve the patient for a period of time and then add in normal food constituents one by one. In this way, a more precise picture of the patient's food allergy profile is obtained. In general terms, I do not think this is necessary. A good observer may well manage to pick out for herself or himself those foods that cause problems.

Alternative medicine

Most conventional doctors have a healthy scepticism about alternative medicine. Presumably, this is based partly on the fact that to become a specialist takes twenty years of intense study, work, and experience. How can somebody 'put up their plate' without any training in basic medicine? On the other hand, according to the law of supply and demand, it must be said that many patients—very many patients—obtain help from various forms of alternative medicine. I think that, if I had lupus, I would try everything, including any form of alternative medicine, provided it was not 'daylight robbery' as far as costs were concerned. I therefore never say no to any patient who asks whether I would advise trying homeopathy, acupuncture, etc. Very many of my patients who are extremely good observers undoubtedly find these various forms of therapy beneficial. A danger of alternative medicine is the total stopping of all drugs which some patients feel is necessary, and we have had a number of catastrophes ('Friday night admissions') where patients have been wooed by one or other form of alternative medicine and have decided to stop their drugs immediately. Most patients are intelligent enough to choose for themselves whether or not an alternative medicine claim is appropriate in their case. Beware of media overkill. Unfortunately, for every one article or radio programme on conventional medicine, such as lupus and its management, there are possibly a dozen on various forms of alternative medicine. Perhaps one day the pendulum will swing back towards the real world a little more, and those who publicize newer forms of alternative medicine may temper their enthusiasm with a tendency towards more scientific appraisal.

Physiotherapy

Physiotherapy (including hydrotherapy) plays a central role in the treatment of patients with muscle and joint problems. Fortunately, the majority of lupus patients do not suffer severe arthritis, but many develop tendon and muscle problems which are sufficiently troublesome to need physiotherapy treatment. The golden rule, in terms of rest and exercise in arthritis patients, is when the joints and muscles are inflamed (continuously painful, swollen, or tender) the treatment is rest; once the 'acute' phase is over, or the patient is responding to medical therapy, the aim is gradual rehabilitation through exercise programmes. Lupus is now taught to physiotherapists and is fortunately becoming recognized as an important illness.

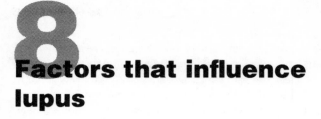

8 Factors that influence lupus

Introduction

There are a number of factors that influence the course of lupus. These include stress, certain drugs and chemicals, hormone changes, and ultraviolet light (i.e. from the sun). Despite these factors, the vast majority of patients flare for unknown reasons.

Factors influencing lupus
- Stress
- Drugs
- Hormones
- Ultraviolet light
- Viruses

Stress

Stress often has a dramatic effect on the course of lupus. Very many patients quite clearly pinpoint the onset of their clinical disease to some form of stress or a period of particularly difficult home or work life. I had one patient who suffered two dramatic flares of lupus following two bereavements in her family. There is some scientific basis for this clinical observation. It is known that acute stress has a marked effect on the immune system and studies of bereavement, for example, have themselves shown that the immune system is affected by stress, such as the grief associated with the loss of a family member. For milder and less dramatic flares, stress may also be a provocative factor.

It is impossible to get rid of stress. It is part of normal life and, although it is advisable for the patient to know stress may influence the disease, it is hard to predict that lupus may improve by removing that source of stress. For the lupus patient this often presents a difficult problem. For example, changing a job because it is difficult and stressful may, on the one hand, help the illness. On the other hand, there is a real danger that it is the lupus itself which is causing the patient's illness, and contributing to the difficulties in the job. Making a major career choice inappropriately could cause more stress. In general, it pays to assess the lupus first to see if this can be improved medically, before making other major decisions.

Drugs

Certain drugs are known to exacerbate lupus. These include sulphonamides and sulphur-containing drugs, such as the antibiotic Septrin, and occasionally, penicillin. It has been suggested that other chemicals, in particular, nitrate-containing chemicals may exacerbate lupus. The evidence is not strong but it is still an important subject for research and one which I think will produce interesting leads over the next few years. Obviously, food additives or the chemical sprays in agriculture and industry, for example, may play a part in exacerbating lupus and I think it is necessary for all of us looking after lupus patients to study these factors.

Hormones

Hormonal changes may affect lupus; the most dramatic being immediately after having a baby when the very rapid hormone changes seem to coincide with a tendency to flares of the disease. In women, the premenstrual period is a particularly important time for lupus flares and, in those patients with grumbling or active disease, it is not uncommon for the disease to become markedly worse in the three to four days before menstruation. In some patients, we even advocate a slight increase in therapy during this period and a small number of my patients on steroids, for example, manage to maintain their dose at a lower level during the first three weeks of the menstrual cycle and increase slightly during the premenstrual period.

Ultraviolet light

It has been known for many years that ultraviolet (UV) light may cause a flare of lupus. The mechanism by which this happens is not known, though it is interesting that the chemical DNA is altered by UV light into a different type of chemical which is highly allergic. It may well be that the effect of UV light on skin alters the skin DNA. Whether this is important or not, it is certain that some lupus patients pinpoint the onset of the disease to a holiday in the sun.

Advice regarding sun protection is, however, not entirely straight-forward. First, not all lupus patients are sun-sensitive. My own esti-mate is that approximately half of my patients have clear-cut histories of photosensitivity, the other half being able to go on holiday with impunity. Second, the tendency to sun-sensitivity may well vary. Patients who, during the active phase of their disease are very sun-sensitive, may well get over this problem. Unfortunately, there are no good scientific methods of pinpointing whether a person is UV-sensi-tive or not, and, although the patient will soon find out by trial and error, it pays to be vigilant. I would certainly advocate the use of sun-screens for any patient initially diagnosed as having lupus who is planning to be in the sun for some time. It is even more important to avoid excess direct UV exposure, especially during the middle of the day. The car is one place where UV exposure often occurs over a period of hours, even through the car window, and it is important to wear long sleeves and, if necessary, a hat. Having said this, my own feeling is that the story of sun-sensitivity in lupus has been slightly exaggerated. Many of my patients who are initially diagnosed as having lupus feel that they are condemned to a life indoors. This is certainly not the case and the true picture is usually found out through trial and error and over time. There are a number of photo-sensitivity studies going on throughout the world and it may well be possible one day to predict more precisely those skins which are more photosensitive. Until that time, take care in the sun!

Be vigilant in the sun!

Other factors

As the majority of lupus patients have no idea why the disease should suddenly become apparent, a considerable amount of research has been undertaken into trying to pinpoint other risk factors. Certainly virus infections, such as influenza, may well exacerbate lupus and it has long been the belief that many researchers that lupus itself is actually triggered by a virus or a group of viruses. As mentioned above, a whole variety of chemicals have been implicated—in one published study, lipstick, because of the pigments used, was proposed as a reason for female lupus patients outnumbering males!

Immunization

The question of immunization is a difficult one. There is no doubt that one or two patients have clearly had a flare of their disease following vaccination and immunization. And it is a fact that injected protein can certainly stimulate the immune response—possibly in an exaggerated way in the lupus patient. This is certainly an area where more studies are needed. My advice is to limit immunization to the absolute minimum requirement for the particular country visited, recognizing that in some countries, immunization or vaccination is mandatory for certain diseases.

Geography

The studies of lupus around the world (the epidemiology of lupus) have not thrown any light on what factors trigger the disease. The ratio of females to males—nine to one—is almost identical throughout Africa, Asia, Europe, and other continents. The disease has not convincingly thrown up pockets of a very high incidence of lupus—a finding which tends to argue against local infections or other triggering factors.

Part VI

What about pregnancy?

9
Lupus in pregnancy

Introduction

How times have changed! Only twenty-five years ago, a survey showed that the majority of patients had been advised by one or other of their doctors against embarking on pregnancy. Lupus, a potentially fatal disease, it was said, would get worse during pregnancy and the chances of a successful birth were minimal. Now, in the weekly lupus pregnancy clinic at St Thomas' Hospital, London, we appear to have rapidly increasing numbers of successful lupus pregnancies—which is mirrored worldwide. Indeed, a considerable amount of research is being conducted and international symposia are being held around the world on lupus in pregnancy.

Despite the interest and research in hormone levels in lupus, in clinical practice menstrual periods are, for the most part, normal. However, when the patient is ill it is not uncommon for periods to stop, sometimes for many months. Likewise, conception in most patients is not a particular problem and lupus is not one of the major causes of infertility in either females or males. Furthermore, contraception is safe in the majority of lupus patients. Clearly there are worries about the high dosage estrogen pill, especially in patients who have migraines or clotting problems associated with antiphospholipid antibodies (see Chapter 15). But again, a survey of our own patients showed that the same proportion of females with lupus were taking the various oral contraceptives as in non-lupus populations and there certainly did not appear to be any obvious increased risk of side effects. My own advice, therefore, when asked about the 'pill' is that, provided the lupus itself is not severe, low-dosage estrogen ('mini-pill') oral contraception is safe. For the most part, pregnancy in lupus patients is relatively uncomplicated. If one assumes that lupus is a life-long disease—you are born with it—then it is clear that many thousands of lupus patients have had successful pregnancies without knowing they have the disease itself.

Pregnancy and lupus: common questions

- Will the disease flare?
- Which drugs should be stopped?
- How can a miscarriage be avoided?
- Will the baby be affected?
- Is breast-feeding possible?

Does the disease flare in pregnancy?

Each year we publish our experience on pregnancy in lupus. When we observe our lupus patients during each of the three-month (trimester) periods of pregnancy, we find that flares of lupus appear to be slightly increased in the second and third trimesters, as well as the puerperium (during the first few months after delivery). In general, the flares are mild and easily treated.

The puerperium

This is the time—the first few months after delivery—when things can go wrong in lupus. Indeed, we sometimes see patients in the first two to three days after delivery suddenly developing the first manifestations of obvious disease. This is one of the most important reasons for combined lupus pregnancy clinics. The patients need very careful, regular monitoring during this critical time when hormone changes are dramatic and when the immune system is severely affected. Our advice, therefore, to patients is that they are monitored during pregnancy, but more frequently after delivery.

Management of the sick pregnant lupus patient

A number of our patients have relatively active lupus during pregnancy and, clearly, hospital management may be needed at certain periods for these individuals. A rise in blood pressure is one of the most common problems, especially in those patients who have mild to moderate kidney disease. In the past, kidney disease was considered a total exclusion as far as pregnancy was concerned, but even this is now no longer the case. Blood pressure can become extremely difficult to manage, however, and requires careful monitoring. Fortunately, modern drugs for blood pressure are much more effective.

Drugs in pregnancy

It comes as something of a surprise to many patients that the majority of drugs used in lupus are in fact safe in pregnancy. This is certainly true of steroids which, it can be argued, are probably the only 'natural' drug used in lupus; steroids being a product of the adrenal gland. In some patients with active lupus, high doses of steroids, even 40 mg daily, have been used during pregnancy. Clearly, this high dose regime poses problems (obviously, the weight gain produced by steroids is especially important to monitor during pregnancy) and it is fortunate that only a small minority of patients require large doses at this time. It was once considered that antimalarials could not be used during pregnancy but we, as well as colleagues in America, are building up data to suggest that hydroxychloroquine (e. g. Plaquenil) can be used safely in pregnancy. For patients with more severe illness, particularly kidney diseases, drugs such as azathioprine may be needed. The data, perhaps surprisingly, show that azathioprine does not pose a major threat, to either mother or baby. When we last checked for pregnancies some years ago in Britain 1500 women had had successful pregnancies while on azathioprine!

As far as other drugs are concerned, each one must be carefully noted by the doctor and checked in the drug formulary or with the manufacturers to make sure there are no adverse effects reported in pregnancy. One drug which is ruled out in pregnancy is warfarin (coumarin), an anticoagulant used in those patients with clotting disorders. The reason for this is that warfarin taken through pregnancy has been reported as clearly producing damage to the fetus. Even here, there are exceptions to the rule. Warfarin is toxic to the fetus in early pregnancy. In rare cases where severe blood-clotting problems continue through pregnancy, warfarin is occasionally substituted for heparin in the later stages of pregnancy.

Early miscarriage

The second problem for the lupus patient in pregnancy (the first being a danger of a flare after delivery) is that some patients suffer miscarriage. We now know that one of the ways in which lupus can first show itself is in a patient giving a history of recurrent sponta-neous abortion, often around three to five months. In the last fifteen years one of the major advances in research in lupus has been the recognition that the reason for this is thrombosis (blocking by a blood clot) of the very small placental blood vessels feeding the fetus. When these small vessels clot, the placenta withers and the fetal blood supply becomes inadequate with resultant miscarriage. Happily, a number of these patients are now being treated successfully using ways of thinning the blood. This will be discussed in Chapter 15, on the antiphospholipid (Hughes') syndrome.

Is the baby affected by lupus?

There is no increased risk of major congenital (or other) illnesses in the offspring of lupus parents. There is certainly a slightly increased family history of lupus, but this does not constitute a strong enough reason to advise against pregnancy in those wishing to have a family. There is, however, one (fortunately very rare) problem which is attracting a lot of research interest. In about 1 in 1000 lupus patients, the child is born with congenital heart block—basically a slow pulse— a rate of 40 beats per minute or so. Although this is usually not life-threatening, it can affect the heart function in the small child, and even affect growth. In the more severely involved children, a pace-maker is required. This defect is known to be associated with the pres-ence of an antibody—anti-Ro (see Chapter 4). Anti-Ro occurs in a quarter of all lupus patients and the mathematics show therefore that, even if anti-Ro is present, the chances of congenital heart block are still less than 1 in 250. It is thought that the Ro-antibody, crossing from the mother's bloodstream, sticks to the electrical conducting tissue in the baby's heart, and causes an abnormal heartbeat rate.

Rashes in the baby

An interesting phenomenon (very rare, I have only seen a dozen or so cases myself) is a lupus-like rash which occurs in the first few weeks on the baby. This rash may mimic adult lupus, and is given the name 'neonatal lupus'. It is now known to be due to passage of the mother's antibody (especially anti-Ro) across the placenta. This antibody then sticks to and causes inflammation in the baby's skin. Although alarming for the mother, the rash is usually mild and disappears when the antibody has disappeared from the child's blood. The mother can be reassured that this is not a sign of present or future lupus in her child.

Breast-feeding

Breast-feeding is not a problem in the majority of lupus' patients. Clearly, some of the drugs used in lupus that are capable of being carried across in breast milk may be potentially toxic to the child and would have to be checked on an individual basis. For the patient on steroids, breast-feeding poses no problem as far as the baby is concerned.

10
Genetics and lupus: will my child get it?

In every large lupus clinic, there are patients who have a clear-cut family history of the disease—two sisters, for example, or a mother and daughter. Now that the disease has 'come out into the open', there are clearly more families in whom a lupus link exists. For example, the aunt who has kidney disease, or the distant cousin who has arthritis and rashes, may well have variants of the disease or more classical lupus itself.

Dozens of studies have been carried out looking at family histories of lupus and these studies have to be interpreted with great caution. If the studies are simply the results of questionnaires sent out, for example, to lupus societies, then the results have to be viewed with even more caution. In any questionnaire, there is always a bias towards increasing the prevalence of the disease within that family—obviously when a disease is recognized as being present in a member of the family, then other possibly distant features may become recognized in family discussions.

More careful studies, including blood test samples, for example, have also been carried out throughout the world and there is no doubt that a small but definite genetic tendency exists. The most common finding in clinical studies of this sort has been the presence of an increased number of patients with very mild or minimal lupus amongst the relatives of patients attending lupus clinics. Even more specifically, there is an increased number of patients' relatives with various antibodies who have no clinical features of the disease but simply the blood test markers for the disease. About thirty years ago, blood testing really grew into a science, with the need for more precise 'fingerprint' testing for organ transplants, etc. A number of diseases were found to be associated with various blood groups. The most classical of these was the disease, ankylosing spondylitis, a condition where the spine becomes stiff, which was strongly associated with a rare white cell blood group—HLA B27 (normally found in 5% of the population of Britain, but found in 95% of ankylosing spondylitis patients). Almost all the major diseases have since been similarly studied for evidence of an association with tissue type, and it was no surprise that there was a statistical association in lupus with certain blood groups, notably HLA B8 and DR3. From the research point of view, an even more interesting finding was made—the association with a rare 'complement' abnormality. If one looks at the sixth chromosome, the sites of many of the genetic markers are now known, and among these, a marker for the development of one of a series of blood proteins called complement can be seen (see Chapter 3). Some 80% of lupus patients have an absent or 'C4 null' genetic marker for complement. Although too cumbersome to be used as a screening test for lupus, this finding was of interest to researchers in lupus for one major reason—complement is one of the protective mechanisms against outside invasion by, for example, viruses. A subtle abnormality of complement might well provide a partial explanation for the development of lupus in these genetically susceptible individuals.

Genetics is one of the fastest growing subjects in medicine. For example, it is now possible to pinpoint genes that:

(1) affect responses to infection,

(2) affect the degree of inflammation,

(3) affect the possibility of having different types of connective tissue (joint) diseases.

And there are dozens more.

In the not too distant future, with the complete mapping of the human genome (the DNA code print-out), it may even be possible to predict the statistical chance of developing a whole range of diseases at birth—a daunting prospect in some ways!

Part VII

Lupus does not only affect young women

11
Lupus in childhood

Introduction

Not unnaturally, the worry and fear created when a diagnosis of lupus is first made in an adult is multiplied many times when that diagnosis is given to a child. A first glance at the textbooks and their descriptions of lupus would make any parent believe that their child had little hope of surviving into adult life. This is wrong. The prognosis in children is no different from that in adults. Obviously, because children are different in the ways they show their illness, diagnosis may sometimes prove difficult, especially as lupus is rare below the age of twelve.

Peak age of onset

Lupus is relatively rare before the onset of menstrual periods. Equally, it is rare in all children under the age of twelve. After that age the graph goes up exponentially. Nevertheless, exceptions always occur and I have patients of two, three, and four years of age.

The earliest form of lupus is not 'true' lupus. It is 'neonatal lupus', a condition of the new-born discussed in Chapter 9 (Lupus in pregnancy). Very occasionally, patients with anti-Ro antibodies give birth to children who, during the first few weeks of life, develop a rash very like lupus. This is not the true disease but is thought to be due to the effect of the mother's antibody which has crossed the placenta and is circulating in the child. As the level of the mother's antibody slowly subsides, so the rash subsides in the baby.

Many analyses have now been carried out on groups of children with lupus and, in the medium- to long-term follow-up series (now mostly into adult life), the same mixture of patterns of lupus emerges.

Lupus children do not, in general terms, have a worse or a better prognosis, a greater or a lesser chance of kidney disease, or any differences in the pattern of their immune response. In the research section, I will be discussing a rare group of individuals who have a deficiency in one of their blood proteins called 'complement'. Some of these individuals develop lupus at an early age and so-called 'complement-deficiency states' may well be a predisposing factor to the development of lupus in, occasionally, very young patients.

The onset of periods

There are major hormone changes in girls around the time of the first menstrual period and it is perhaps not surprising, in view of what has been said earlier, that this is the time that the diagnosis of lupus first starts to be made in real numbers. It is rather unusual to have a classical butterfly rash (which would make the diagnosis easily apparent), but more common are the rather non-specific signs such as tiredness, failure to do well at school, aches and pains, headaches, recurring 'glandular fever', and so on. Obviously, these are such non-specific and common features that lupus, to put it in its true context, must be considered a very 'small-print' cause of these common features to confront the family doctor. Perhaps this is one of the reasons why there is a slight increase in the number of diagnosed cases of lupus in the relatives and daughters of lupus patients, for example. Perhaps they are more aware of the disease and put that much more pressure on their doctors to consider a diagnosis of lupus.

Should I have my child tested?

To summarize, lupus is not a very strongly inherited disease. Statistically, there really is no reason why all the offspring of lupus patients should have blood tests. This being said, as in all the auto-immune diseases, there is a niggling, though slight risk. In my experience, unless there are symptoms in the children, testing before the early teens is not very fruitful and the results are almost invariably negative. After that, the tests become far more useful. My own advice, therefore, is that if a parent has a child with symptoms which really have defied diagnosis, then yes, the antinuclear antibody (ANA) test should certainly be done. It is cheap and reasonably sensitive. If, in the opinion of the observant mother, the child really does have features which strongly suggest lupus, she should insist that her doctor has her child tested.

Treatment

There are no major differences from the treatment used in adults. For acute or major lupus, steroids are almost always used. Steroids in childhood have the major drawback of slowing growth, and efforts are intensified to keep the dose to a minimum in this age group.

Following data obtained in other diseases, such as asthma and Still's disease, where a vast amount of experience has been accumulated, many doctors advocate the use of 'alternate-days' steroids. There is some data to suggest that this allows better growth, though it must be said that there is no absolute proof of this.

12
Lupus in males

Although lupus is uncommon in males, it does not differ in any major way from the pattern of lupus in females. Also, rather mysteriously, despite the fact that lupus is a predominantly female disease, there is absolutely nothing to suggest that males with the disease are in any way less than 'male'. They have normal sperm counts, raise families, and even, in the case of one of my patients, become amateur boxing champions! The clinical investigation of lupus in males has been something of an obsession for those of us who study lupus. Despite the feeling that the disease might somehow be different in its format, this has never been proved to be the case. Thus, the same percentages of patients have kidney disease, rashes, and so on.

Hormone effects (see Chapter 21 on Research) are undoubtedly important. It is said that lupus is nine times more common in females than in males. However, if one looks at children under the age of twelve, for example, the ratio is much closer (three girls to one boy). Likewise, in the sixty-year-olds, the ratio again is something like three to one. In the mid twenties to mid thirties, the ratio of female to male approaches thirty to one.

Causes of lupus in the male

The same causes apply to males as to females. Occasionally, there are males with a family history of lupus, and others in whom extreme sun exposure has apparently triggered the disease. In one or two of my male patients, it is possible that certain drugs, such as antibiotics, triggered the disease, and this raises the rather difficult question of whether, in these patients, the disease was initially 'true' lupus or 'drug-induced' lupus.

Treatment

At the present time, treatment of lupus in males is exactly the same as that used in females. If male hormone treatment has a beneficial effect on patients (and there is a sprinkling of research evidence that this might be the case), then there may well be future directions for studies of newer hormone-related treatments in males with lupus.

13
Lupus in the older patient

Recently, a young research fellow working in my department, proudly produced for me a study done in my clinic on 'lupus in the elderly'. Her definition of 'elderly' was fifty!

There are many facts but a lot of unknowns in this area:

1. It is a fact that lupus is much less common in older patients.
2. It is extremely unusual for a major and serious flare, such as a new case of kidney disease, to develop at the age of forty-five or older.
3. In the female, when the menopause occurs, and the hormone changes that accompany it are manifested, it is normal for the blood tests to become less positive and even revert to negative.

Unfortunately, this is not the full story. There are undoubtedly patients who still continue to suffer considerable clinical problems (e.g. joint pains) after the menopause, and there are a number of lupus patients in any clinic aged sixty or more who still have clinical symptoms.

Is it lupus or is it something else?

The importance of definition

Many patients who are diagnosed as having lupus at the age of, say, fifty, in fact have Sjögren's syndrome (see Chapter 17) with blood tests such as positive anti-nuclear antibody. These, on first impression, suggest a diagnosis of lupus. To be precise—and it is important to be precise—this is not lupus in its true sense. Sjögren's syndrome is a grumbling but benign disease and therefore deserves to be distinguished from systemic lupus erythematosus (SLE). There are many other causes of positive anti-nuclear (ANA) tests (see Chapter 4). Another scenario is the patient who has had mild lupus for many years, and for some reason at this age has a flare of joint pains. Certainly, this is still compatible with the diagnosis of lupus but, again, it is usually a diagnosis that implies a good prognosis.

Joint pains

Arthritis is the major feature of lupus and lupus-like diseases in older patients. This varies from the occasional joint pains to the full-blown swollen joints resembling rheumatoid arthritis (see Chapters 17 and 18). Whatever the underlying diagnosis, the treatment is pragmatic and based on the severity of the arthritis. Thus, for 'mild Sjögren's' with joint pains, non-steroidal anti-inflammatory drugs and anti-malarials may be sufficient, while for those with severe 'rheumatoid' disease (see Chapter 18), stronger drugs, such as methotrexate, may be required. General information on these medications is given in Chapter 5. Fortunately, patients over the age of fifty often respond to very low doses of steroids, such as 5 mg daily. Obviously at this age, the risk of osteoporosis (bone softening) becomes a major problem as a side effect of steroid usage.

Skin rashes

Discoid lupus (see Chapter 16) is the major skin rash which continues to cause problems in the fifty year olds and over. Problems are sometimes compounded by the presence of continuing joint pains, headaches, depression and other features of more general illness. Nevertheless, these patients are very amenable to treatment and, if possible, should always attend clinic specializing in lupus and its variants.

The antiphospholipid (Hughes') syndrome

Our knowledge of this relatively new syndrome (see Chapter 15) is growing quickly. We do not know, however, how significant a cause it is or subtle 'brain' symptoms, such as depression, tiredness, memory impairment, lack of attention, etc. Studies are now going to throughout the world using sophisticated techniques, such as MRI (magnetic resonance imaging—brain scanning), in patients with antiphospholipid antibodies to see whether very localized and small thrombosis might have been far more common than we had previously anticipated. This is a field where research really will directly help not only our knowledge of lupus, but also our patients.

Part VIII
Lupus-like diseases

14

Mixed connective tissue disease

This cumbersome title confuses both doctors and patients alike. Yet it is an important disease, in many ways similar to lupus and to all intents and purposes, classifiable as lupus.

Disease history

In the early 1970s, the use of various antibody tests showed that there were different types of lupus, just as doctors and patients had long recognized. In 1973, Dr Sharp and colleagues in America described a disease or syndrome which was like lupus but differed in one major respect; it rarely produced kidney disease. It was given the title 'mixed' because it had some of the features of lupus, as well as some of the features of another disease, 'scleroderma' (see Chapter 18), and occasionally, just to give it a real 'mongrel' image, some patients developed inflammation of the muscles, 'myositis'.

Mixed connective tissue disease (MCTD) is characterized by four major features:

1. Raynaud's phenomenon—very cold tips of fingers and toes.

2. Prominent arthritis—'sausage fingers'.

3. The absence (or rarity) of many of the more general features of lupus, such as kidney disease.

4. A specific blood test. Although 'classical' lupus patients have anti-DNA antibodies, patients with 'mixed' connective tissue disease do not. They do, invariably, have in their blood another antibody—the so-called 'anti RNP'. See Chapters 3 and 4 for details of blood tests.

Raynaud's phenomenon

This is where the fingers suddenly become cold and white. Classically, fingers go through the colours red, white, and blue—or, more correctly, they first turn white (often suddenly and dramatically and for no apparent reason, though more usually precipitated by cold). After a period of whiteness, the fingers then turn bluish and finally, when circulation returns, they may glow and even pulsate. Oddly, one or two fingers only may be affected. Raynaud's phenomenon (named after the doctor who first described it) is a common problem and is not usually associated with any underlying illness. There are many thousands of individuals throughout the world who suffer from it.

It can, however, be a manifestation of a number of diseases, notably, the group of 'connective tissue diseases', of which lupus is a member. Lupus patients themselves often suffer from mild to moderate Raynaud's. The Raynaud's phenomenon in mixed connective tissue disease (MCTD), however, is very much prominent and reminiscent of that seen in scleroderma (see Chapter 18). Unfortunately, it is very difficult to treat and other than taking very careful precautions before going out in cold weather (some patients even use electrically heated gloves), there is no ideal drug at the present time.

Arthritis

In mixed connective tissue disease, the picture is much more reminiscent of rheumatoid arthritis with much swelling, especially in the fingers. Characteristically, the fingers may become 'sausage-like'. The swelling may become troublesome, severe, and persistent and these patients will often resort to stronger antirheumatic drugs such as methotrexate (see Chapter 5). Other joints may also be involved in MCTD but one of the odd characteristics of the disease is its propensity to affect fingers more than most other joints.

Other manifestations

Occasionally, there may be a true inflammation of the muscles, with muscle pain as well as muscle weakness. In some patients, this is the first manifestation of the disease. When other organs are inflamed, MCTD poses a diagnostic 'grey area', sometimes referred to by doctors as 'overlap syndrome'. Pleurisy, for example, can be prominent and one or other of the more general manifestations of lupus certainly can occur. Fortunately, kidney disease is rare.

Treatment

Although general management of these diseases will be discussed later, there are some particular problems in the management of mixed connective tissue disease. Because it is less 'life-threatening' than some of the other diseases discussed in this book, it follows that more conservative treatment should be the rule. Yet many patients with MCTD seem to require low to moderate doses of steroids for many years. Attempts at weaning patients off steroids are often difficult and even the use of higher doses of antimalarials and other antirheumatic drugs is sometimes unsuccessful. We have, like others, been using the drug methotrexate (see Chapter 5), which has proved revolutionary in the management of rheumatoid arthritis, and in some of our patients on methotrexate there has been improvement in the joints. Medications, such as nifedipine (a drug widely used for circulation disorders), are used for the treatment of Raynaud's phenomenon, but, as mentioned, they are less than perfect. Patients and doctors alike impatiently await advances in the treatment of Raynaud's phenomenon.

Conclusion

Mixed connective tissue disease, despite its problematical name, is a very specific condition, causing cold fingers and joint pains. Although it does not usually produce life-threatening complications, it is often painful and requires frequent monitoring of treatment.

15

The antiphospholipid (Hughes') syndrome— 'sticky' blood

Introduction

In 1983, we described a group of lupus patients with a disorder characterized by blood clotting, both in arteries and veins. These patients also had a tendency to recurrent miscarriages and more widespread problems notably a danger of strokes. This syndrome has become known as 'sticky blood'—or Hughes' syndrome—or more prosaically, as the antiphospholipid syndrome (APS).

Phospholipids are the chemicals contained in the membrane of the cells of the body, including the important lining cells of blood vessels, and the membrane of platelets—the agents involved in clotting. Our original studies concentrated on lupus patients, some of whom have APS, but it quickly became apparent that many more patients— indeed, the vast majority of patients with the antiphospholipid syndrome (or Hughes' syndrome as it is now sometimes called) do not have lupus.

This discovery has been important to those within the lupus field for two main reasons. First, it has shown that not all the features of lupus are due to inflammation of blood and blood vessels—other mechanisms, such as thrombosis, may be important. Second, the discovery changes our thinking in terms of the management (i.e. with the use of anti-clotting drugs) of some of our patients who might previously have been treated with steroids or other anti-inflammatory medications. Putting it simply, there are two major types of disease process in lupus: inflammation and thrombosis, each of which has a different mechanism and appropriately different treatment.

Clinical features

Any vein may clot in severe cases of the Hughes' syndrome. Some patients first show signs of the disease in their teens with a leg vein thrombosis (occasionally associated with the contraceptive pill). In others, there may be a clot in the arm with swelling or thrombosis of internal veins such as those connected to the liver, digestive system, or in the lungs. Much more sinister is the danger of arterial thrombosis. Some patients with the syndrome first present dramatically with thrombosis of, for example, a leg or an arm artery. Some patients develop thrombosis of an internal organ, such as the heart or adrenal glands, or even the eye or brain. As in lupus, any organ is potentially at risk of thrombosis in this syndrome and, in many ways, it is a far more dangerous disease than more classical lupus.

Brain involvement

One of the common features of these patients has been a tendency to thrombosis in the brain—varying from minor strokes to permanent and crippling strokes. The very minor thromboses produce headaches, visual disturbances, and, occasionally, more subtle disorders such as those associated with movement (e.g. chorea—St Vitus' dance). We have noticed a strong association with recurrent epilepsy in these patients.

Diagnosing and managing this disease is a matter of balance and is of critical importance. It is very hard to know whether a patient with minor or subtle headaches is likely to develop a major thrombosis; my own feeling is that one cannot be cautious enough when dealing with this syndrome. Fortunately, in the majority of patients who have had a blood clot and who have been started appropriately on anticoagulant treatment, all symptoms of the disease have disappeared and the beneficial effect is often dramatic.

The signs and symptoms of this syndrome, although sometimes life-threatening, are generally more subtle—especially some of the 'brain' symptoms. These can include headaches, sometimes with visual disturbances, such as flashing lights, loss of concentration, and memory loss. In some patients, the problem can be very specific, such as the severe inability to remember their shopping list. Two examples, seen in patients of mine, are shown in the box.

> **Case 1**
>
> A 35-year-old woman, the champion of her village darts team, suddenly found that she could no longer accurately hit the correct numbers.
>
> **Case 2**
>
> A well-known 50-year-old sculptress became unable to recognize three-dimensional shapes. She was unable to convert to clay, for example, the shape of a given object, such as a coca cola bottle.

Clearly, neurologists recognize such specific examples as being due to problems in very localized parts of the brain.

In the case of the antiphospholipid syndrome (APS), these defects are due to disturbances in brain circulation resulting from 'thickness' or 'clottiness' of the blood. Perhaps a suitable analogy is the car engine, when the gas or petrol mixture is far too rich. This clearly identifiable problem is going to prove to be a major advance in diagnosis and treatment, not only in lupus, but in many other branches of medicine.

Low platelets

One of the slightly odd features of the disease is that, while it is mainly a thrombotic disease, occasionally the total platelet levels can be reduced—a condition known as 'thrombocytopenia'. Some of our patients have acute drops in platelet levels. More commonly, others fluctuate with borderline results. The normal platelet count is above 150 000 per cm^2 but a number of our patients get along nicely with platelet counts between 30 000 and 80 000. In theory, the danger of having a low platelet count is bleeding. In practice, this is rare unless there is an accident or laceration—most doctors monitor patients with borderline platelet counts, without necessarily stepping in with drugs.

Heart valve disease

Another unusual aspect of APS is that occasionally patients develop abnormalities of the valve of the heart, partially from a blood clot around the valve. As usual, the first sign of this is either shortness of breath or a murmur heard on a clinical examination. Usually this is benign. Indeed, long before these clinical signs are apparent, minor degrees of valve involvement can be picked up on an echocardiogram (heart echo scan). Sometimes, however, there is a more severe deterioration in the heart valve—very occasionally requiring heart valve surgery.

Pregnancy

As mentioned in Chapter 9, patients with antiphospholipid antibodies (aPL) suffer thrombosis of the placenta and recurrent miscarriages. Until this syndrome was described, the cause of the recurrent abortions seen in some lupus patients was unknown. APS has become a major syndrome in the practice of obstetrics. If one takes all women attending a pregnancy clinic who suffer from recurrent miscarriages, the percentage who will have this potentially treatable mechanism is significant—in some studies, up to 25%. The treatment is with an anticoagulant, often low dose aspirin but more often, in patients who have had previous medical problems (especially thrombosis), with other types of anticoagulant (see Chapter 6).

Conclusion

The antiphospholipid (Hughes') syndrome is a major breakthrough. It has opened up different ways of thinking about lupus, as well as treating it. More importantly, its discovery has created a new perspective on common clotting disorders such as strokes and heart attacks.

16
Discoid lupus

Introduction

This skin disease is the oldest historical form of lupus and, in many ways, is different from classical lupus. Although discoid disease is less life-threatening, it can pose major problems as far as the skin is concerned and often creates far greater damage to the skin than the rashes of classical lupus.

Features

Characteristically, discoid disease consists of a rash on the cheeks and nose, but also on the scalp and elsewhere in the body. This rash can be disfiguring and sometimes scarring—unlike that of classical lupus. There is thickening of the skin and a scaliness, which often becomes red and 'angry'. Scalp involvement (including itchiness, redness, and peeling) may be very prominent, and patches of baldness may occur. In the more, severe cases there is widespread scalp involvement and a marked loss of hair; fortunately this is rare. Involvement of the fingers and feet can be prominent and the skin can become cracked and painful. The nails are frequently involved, becoming brittle, fragile, and curled (in some ways resembling the abnormal nails in the skin disease, psoriasis). The skin patches often affect the ears, especially the external ear canal, and in some patients there are mouth ulcers inside the lips. In contrast to classical 'systemic' lupus erythematosus (SLE), discoid disease can affect patients of all ages and frequently occurs in the late sixties.

Systemic disease

Approximately 5% of patients with discoid lupus at some stage develop more widespread disease, classifiable as systemic lupus.

Although this overlap is small, it is nevertheless significant, and patients with discoid lupus, who feel unwell or develop other clinical problems, should be investigated for SLE.

Dry eyes

A proportion of patients with discoid lupus also develop dryness of the eyes and mouth. The condition as Sjögren's syndrome (see Chapter 17). Physicians are often unaware of the association between discoid lupus and Sjögren's syndrome, but treatment, especially of the dry eyes, can bring considerable relief to patients.

Joint pain

One rather odd feature of 'discoid' lupus is the occasional attack of arthritis. This may be the only other manifestation of the disease (without any internal organ involvement). We have a number of patients in their fifties to seventies who have 'discoid' lupus and a grumbling form of arthritis—in some cases, moderately severe and resembling 'low-grade' rheumatoid arthritis. This subset of lupus patients obviously deserves closer study. However, it is important to remember that these patients rarely have any life-threatening internal disease.

Brain involvement

There is, however, one potentially dangerous problem of 'discoid' lupus. A small number of these patients have antiphospholipid antibodies (aPL) and the clotting disorder (Hughes' syndrome) associated with these antibodies (see Chapter 15). One or two of our discoid patients have developed serious strokes. It is probably wise, therefore, to recommend aPL screening in discoid patients, as well as in systemic lupus patients. In addition to the more florid central nervous diseases, such as strokes, milder, though still troublesome, brain problems, including periods of depression, mental tiredness, and exhaustion are quite frequent in some patients with discoid. These are hard to explain, certainly on the basis of the generally normal blood tests seen in discoid, but there is no doubt that they are real.

Treatment

The antimalarial family of drugs has proved enormously useful in discoid lupus, though sometimes high doses are required. Various steroid ointments are also used and these will be discussed later. In extreme cases, recent data have suggested that the drug thalidomide is useful, though clearly the decision to use this potentially dangerous drug needs to be taken with great care. For more information about medications used, see Chapter 5. Finally, a small number of my patients, with prominent facial scarring from discoid lupus, have had very successful plastic surgery.

Conclusion

Discoid lupus is predominantly a skin form of lupus—often chronic and sometimes scarring, but almost always free from the internal organ disease which distinguishes systemic lupus from discoid lupus.

17
Sjögren's syndrome

Introduction

In many ways, Sjögren's syndrome can be regarded as a mild form of lupus. In 1930, Hendrick Sjögren, a Swedish ophthalmologist, noticed that some of the patients attending his eye clinic suffered from poor tear secretion. In addition, they had dryness of the mouth. More importantly, he noticed that this group of patients with dryness (or 'sicca' syndrome) also had a more widespread rheumatic disease, such as rheumatoid arthritis. The triad now known as Sjögren's syndrome, consists of dry mouth, dry eyes, and a connective tissue disease (most commonly rheumatoid arthritis). We now know that most connective tissue diseases can be associated with Sjögren's syndrome, including systemic lupus, mixed connective tissue disease (MCTD), discoid lupus, and scleroderma. All age groups are affected, though the average age is older than for classical lupus. Sjögren's syndrome is, in many ways, most closely related to lupus; even some of the blood tests (such as the antinuclear antibodies test) overlap.

Indeed, many lupus patients reaching the age of fifty or over, even though the systemic disease settles down, are left with Sjögren's syndrome—troublesome dryness affecting the mucous membranes around the eyes and in the mouth.

Dryness

The eyes are often gritty and scratchy, especially in the morning. Sometimes, there is a photosensitivity to bright light. Somewhat surprisingly, the patient often does not realize that the eyes are dry. The test for dry eyes is a simple one. A strip of blotting paper, several millimetres long, is hooked over the eyelid. In most individuals, this intensely irritating stimulus causes profuse tear secretion—within seconds the blotting paper is wet. In Sjögren's, the blotting paper often remains totally dry, even after waiting for five minutes. There are more 'elaborate' tests for dryness of the eyes, including staining of the conjunctiva with a dye (e. g. Rose-Bengal dye) and slit-lamp examination (the instrument used for viewing the eye) carried out an ophthalmologist.

The mouth may also be dry. This presents considerable problems, not only in swallowing dry food such as biscuits, but obviously in swallowing pills. In time, the absence of normal saliva creates an unhealthy environment and dental decay is prominent in patients with severe sicca syndrome. Regular and good dental treatment is clearly mandatory in patients with this syndrome. The dryness may extend down the back of the throat making swallowing difficult, and some patients find that they are so affected by this, that they have take a jug of water to bed with them at night.

Other mucous membranes of the body may also be dry including the lining of the stomach and the vagina, and in some patients there is not only pain on intercourse but an increased danger of vaginal infections, notably thrush. Luckily, in most lupus patients who have Sjögren's syndrome, the severity of dryness is minimal and the only treatment usually given are artificial tears for the eyes.

Arthritis

Joint pains are common in Sjögren's syndrome. They may vary from mild to medium joint problems seen in lupus patients, through to full-blown rheumatoid arthritis. In other patients, joint pains are absent and such patients (usually referred to as having the 'primary sicca syndrome') are often undiagnosed for many years. A number of patients with Sjögren's syndrome have had a previous diagnosis of ME (myalgic encephalitis), for example.

Other features

As with those with lupus, Sjögren's patients are immunologically overreactive and produce many antibodies. Their globulin level in the blood (the antibody protein) is often high. They are allergic people, as are lupus patients, and have a much higher incidence of allergies to, for example, Septrin, penicillin, and gold (the latter frequently used in the past for arthritis). In some patients, the antibody protein level is extremely high and may even contribute to a clogging up of small blood vessels, leading to small red spots, particularly on the legs, known as 'purpura'. In some of these patients, the purpura become prominent after exercise, such as a game of tennis. Purpura is usually benign and no treatment is required, though in some severe cases it can form a widespread rash, leading to 'pins and needles' in the feet.

Blood tests

Sjögren's patients produce a number of antibodies but, characteristically, they are negative for antibodies against DNA—the hallmark of systemic lupus. The diagnostic antibody test for Sjögren's is the so-called anti-Ro (see Chapter 4 for a more detailed description). Other blood tests seen in lupus are mirrored (to a lesser extent) in Sjögren's (e.g. both have a low white cell count and, occasionally, a low platelet count). Evidence of major internal involvement is unusual. Very rarely, a patient with primary Sjögren's (and it is to be stressed that these are almost invariably not lupus patients with Sjögren's), develops large swellings and even malignancy (lymphoma) in the lymph glands. Usually, this is a very low-grade lymphoma and extremely responsive to treatment. Although these cases are rare, they are important to us in research because they give a clue to a link between the immune diseases and the change to malignant disease in this body system.

Treatment

In most patients with Sjögren's no treatment is required, other than possibly artificial tears (methyl-cellulose eye drops). In others, there may be sufficient joint pains to demand non-steroidal anti-inflammatory drugs (NSAIDs) or antimalarials, and in others, periods on steroids or even immunosuppressives are required (see Chapter 5). However, the prognosis in Sjögren's, is good and significant kidney disease is extremely unusual.

Conclusion

Sjögren's syndrome is common and often not diagnosed or even wrongly labelled as, for example, ME. Most commonly, its features are dry eyes, dry mouth, and joint aches and pains. In many ways it can be regarded as a mild version of lupus, being especially common in patients of forty to sixty years of age.

18

Scleroderma and other connective tissue diseases

Scleroderma

This is a condition where the skin becomes thickened and immobile. It normally begins in the fingers and is associated with severe Raynaud's phenomenon (blood vessel 'spasm' and cold fingers, see Chapter 14). In some patients, it remains confined to the hands and sometimes the feet, but in others it spreads slowly upwards giving a thickened hard, glossy appearance to the skin of the arms, chest, and later the face, especially around the nose and mouth. There may be a similar thickening of internal organs, notably of the oesophagus (the tube through which food passes from the mouth to the stomach), making swallowing difficult and producing symptoms of severe heartburn. Scleroderma is very different from lupus, though in the early stages there may be diagnostic difficulty (e.g. with a patient with mild Raynaud's).

Dermatomyositis

This is an inflammation of the muscles. Normally, there is marked muscle weakness, (e.g. difficulty in standing up from a sitting position or in lifting a heavy book or pan onto a high shelf). Occasionally, there is also muscle tenderness and pain. Although in many patients the disease remains confined to the muscles, in others it involves the skin as well, giving a widespread, purplish skin rash. Sometimes this looks superficially rather like a lupus rash, with red-purple discoloration of the face (especially the eyelids) and V-area of the neck. There may be a red rash on the back of the hands and knuckles. Dermatomyositis is a different disease from lupus, and, although the rash (sometimes very photosensitive) may be similar, the blood tests and further investigations usually quickly differentiate the two diseases.

Wegener's granulomatosis

Because this is a disease that causes inflammation of the blood vessels, it tends to be seen by the same group of doctors who see lupus patients. It is not uncommon in lupus clinics to see patients affected by Wegener's.

Wegener's granulomatosis, is however, totally different. It is a rare, possibly allergic disease causing severe rhinitis and sinusitis (stuffy and dripping nose). This may be so severe that the discharge becomes bloodstained. This chronic thickening in the sinuses affects the sinus areas in the forehead and sometimes behind the eyes, but more seriously, the process can spread to the lungs (e.g. with coughing and shortness of breath) and in more severe cases, to other organs in the body, including the blood vessels, nerves, and kidneys. In the past, this was one of the worst connective tissue diseases, almost invariably fatal; but the advent of the drug cyclophosphamide (see Chapter 5) has reversed this prognosis. These patients are now treated quickly, effectively, and in many cases completely successfully, finally coming off all medication. The cause of Wegener's is unknown, although the similarities to some allergic disease (lung and sinus involvement) suggests that there is an allergic background to the disease. Blood tests and other investigations easily differentiate Wegener's from lupus.

Polyarteritis nodosa

This disease is similar to Wegener's in that it is an inflammatory disease of the blood vessels. However, it is more dramatic with inflammation of the major arteries, often presenting acutely with artery inflammation in the legs (leg pain and difficulty in walking), internal organs (damage to vital internal organs, such as the heart, gut, nerves, etc.), and joint pains. It is a very acute and stormy disease, often life-threatening, but again, if caught early, is completely and totally reversible. Interestingly, once the acute episode has been overcome, it is unusual for this disease to recur. Unlike lupus and Sjögren's syndrome, it affects males more frequently than females. The cause is unknown, but, in some cases, it appears to follow a virus infection—sometimes, the hepatitis virus. Again, it is a different disease from lupus and is easily distinguishable by examination and blood tests.

Rheumatoid arthritis

This is usually a very different disease from lupus. In some patients, however, notably those who have rheumatoid associated with Sjögren's, the blood tests may cause confusion with lupus; and certainly there are many patients in whom the differential diagnosis between rheumatoid and lupus is rather difficult. Characteristically, rheumatoid arthritis, if it continues unabated, causes damage and erosion of the joints, clearly visible on X-ray, whereas lupus does not. Rheumatoid arthritis sometimes produces nodules, especially around the elbows, but lupus rarely does. Finally, rheumatoid arthritis is largely confined to the joints, and serious internal organ involvement such as kidney disease, is unusual.

Still's disease

This name is given to arthritis in childhood, though, just to make life more difficult, Still's disease is occasionally seen in adults. Obviously, there are many types of arthritis in childhood, and Still's probably includes a variety of juvenile diseases which may ultimately develop into, for example, rheumatoid arthritis in some, or lupus in others. There have been major advances in the clinical differentiation at an early stage of Still's, and most physicians dealing with this disease can reasonably accurately pinpoint the direction in which the disease is likely to progress.

Rheumatic fever

This is an acute arthritis which develops in some individuals following a streptococcal sore throat. The disease is becoming rare in Western countries. Nevertheless, it is still often wrongly diagnosed. In less developed countries, where the rapid spread of *Streptococcus* is more frequent, rheumatic fever still poses a major problem. Again, the blood tests normally differentiate it easily from lupus.

Behçet's disease

This is a very common disease in certain communities, notably in some Mediterranean and Middle Eastern countries such as Turkey, Iran, and Iraq. The symptoms are mouth and genital ulcers (often severe and recurrent) and, in some patients, a tendency to arthritis, and more seriously, internal blood vessel problems. Despite these superficial clinical similarities, the diseases are very different indeed and the blood tests clearly distinguish them.

Conclusion

The group of diseases in this chapter resemble lupus only in that they cause joint problems. While many patients with lupus may recall some of these diagnoses being considered early on in the course of their disease, they are usually easily separated, both on clinical grounds and by blood tests.

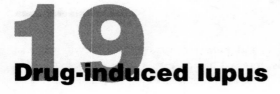

Drug-induced lupus

There are a number of drugs and chemicals that cause a lupus-like disease. Indeed, in some patients drug-induced lupus mimics true lupus so closely that the observations have led to considerable research into chemical and environmental triggers as causes of lupus. The list of drugs which have been implicated in causing drug-induced lupus is very long. Medical students and doctors alike find the list daunting. Fortunately, drug-induced lupus is rare.

> Drug-induced lupus gets better when the offending drug is stopped.

In essence, there are two types of drug reactions. First, there are those drugs that exacerbate true underlying lupus (e.g. Septrin, a sulphonamide-like antibiotic which frequently causes a flare of true lupus in those with the disease). Second, there is a group of drugs that cause skin rashes, joint pains, and other lupus-like phenomena in otherwise healthy individuals (see box). In these patients, the term drug-induced lupus truly applies. Drug-induced lupus has many of the features of lupus and is brought on by a variety of drugs and chemicals. It gets better when the drug is stopped.

Drugs capable of causing Lupus-like disease

- Hydralazine (Blood pressure lowering agent)
- Procainamide (used for heart rhythm problems)
- Sulphasalazine (used in colitis and inrheumatoid)
- Minocycline (antibiotic used for acne)

Similarities to true lupus

The rashes are very similar to those of 'true' lupus, with butterfly rashes, widespread elbow and chest rashes, and vasculitic rashes on the palms and soles of the feet. There may also be hair loss. There are more general features such as malaise, joint pains, pleurisy and lymph gland swelling. Tiredness is a major problem and the disease can be extremely severe.

Differences from true lupus

1. Kidney disease is extremely rare in drug-induced lupus.
2. The blood tests are different. On the whole, drug-induced lupus patients do not produce the same pattern of antibodies (anti-DNA antibodies and antibodies to ENA are absent, see Chapter 4).
3. Most important of all, the disease improves once the offending drug has been stopped.

The true nature of the disease

Some years ago, we studied in detail a group of patients with drug-induced lupus produced by a medicine used for blood pressure—hydralazine. This drug, in moderately high doses, is known to be an occasional cause of drug-induced lupus. Our findings were very interesting. There were three requirements needed to produce the disease. First, the patients had to be slow-metabolizers of hydralazine (i.e. their system could not get rid of the drug very quickly). Second, there was a female preponderance. Third, even more interestingly, there was a blood group association—(DR 4)—a possible genetic factor. Here then is a possible example of 'soil and seed'—the genetic tendency for the disease to lie dormant and be brought out by a chance meeting with a triggering factor such as, in this case, hydralazine.

Treatment

Fortunately, drug-induced lupus is extremely rare. For example, of the 2500 lupus patients in St Thomas' clinic, I currently know of half a dozen in whom the disease was drug-induced. This may well, of course, be an underestimation. Ignorance dictates that we cannot recognize the, presumably, endless list of causes of a flare of lupus. For example, it has come to light that minocycline, an antibiotic widely used for acne, can cause quite an acute form of drug-induced lupus. It is interesting that some of the drugs have chemical similarities, and it has even been suggested that tartrazines—the colouring matter in so many of our foods nowadays, may have a precipitating effect in lupus. On stopping the drugs, the disease quickly gets better—often within weeks or months. So also, do the blood tests. Once the drug is withdrawn the story is usually over. For this reason, it seems likely that drugs and chemicals are potential triggers for an acute attack of the disease, and not the most likely candidates for being the leading cause of true lupus.

Part IX
More about history and research

20 The history of lupus

'Lupus', in one form or another, has been around for at least seven centuries. The word, derived from the Latin for wolf, was used for a variety of skin afflications, 'wolf-bites' affecting the face. Some of these diseases—some infections and skin cancers, for example, untreatable in the past—really did 'eat' into the skin of the face and fully deserved this description. We now know these diseases were very different from the systemic lupus being dealt with here.

Well-known physicians, such as Rogerius in the thirteenth century, and Paracelsus in the early sixteenth century, provided clear descriptions of 'lupus' face lesions. In the early nineteenth century, a number of more precise descriptions led to the realization that different diseases could produce 'lupus-like' skin lesions—the most notable descriptions being those of Cazenave who in 1851–2 reported three different types of lupus, including 'lupus erythemateus'.

Towards the end of the nineteenth century, Dr Payne, a physician at St Thomas' Hospital, London, prescribed the use of antimalarials, not only for skin lupus, but for some of the other effects of the diseases including fever.

In a series of three papers published between 1895 and 1903, the renowned physician William Osler clearly identified that internal organs could be involved, and that lupus could take on a 'systemic' form. His descriptions included involvement of the heart, kidneys, and 'mucous surfaces' (e.g. pleurisy). 'Relapse is a special feature of the disease and attacks may come on month after month or even throughout a long period of years'.

Blood tests

During the 1930s and 1940s, more clinical and pathological studies were published and it became clear that, for the most part, discoid and systemic lupus could be clearly separated.

In 1948, a discovery was made which possibly more than any other, stimulated diagnostic recognition of the disease. Hargreaves, Richmond, and Morton in the journal *Proceedings of the Staff Meetings of the Mayo Clinic* reported:

> In the last two years, we have been observing a phenomenon in our bone marrow preparations which, to our knowledge, has never been described in the literature ... the second cell, which we wish to present, has been called the 'LE cell' in our laboratory because of its frequent appearance in the bone marrow of acute cases of disseminated lupus erythematosus.

The 'LE cell' was in fact a peculiar-looking white blood cell seen under certain circumstances in marrow (and subsequently in blood itself) in some, though not all, lupus patients. In diagnostic testing, the LE cell test (somewhat cumbersome and expensive) was replaced by the ANA (antinuclear antibody test, see Chapter 4). A number of groups, notably Drs Kunkel and Tan in the United States, and Drs Doniach and Holborrow in the UK, spent many years improving the tests.

In 1966, four groups of researchers found that the blood of lupus patients was characterized particularly by antibodies that worked against the 'double helix' DNA, and in 1970–71 the first papers by Drs Pincus, Tan, Christian, and others were published showing that anti-DNA antibody measurement was a sensitive and extraordinarily specific, diagnostic tool for SLE (systemic lupus erythematosus). It was my privilege in 1969–70, as a UK travelling research fellow to Dr Charles Christian's unit in New York, to have been involved in these studies introducing the DNA-binding test to clinical practice.

In the late 1960s and early 1970s, many of the other antibodies were characterized, such as Ro, RNP, etc. (see Chapter 4)—work led by colleagues such as Drs Tan, Reichlin, and Sharpe.

In 1983, my own group described the antiphospholipid syndrome (see Chapter 15). We realized that the presence of antiphospholipid antibodies were associated with a very distinct syndrome—often totally separate from lupus, and associated with artery and vein thrombosis, strokes, miscarriages, and a variety of other features which had, hitherto, been thought to be due to inflammation. The introduction of blood-thinning treatment, rather than, for example, using steroids, has altered our thinking about the disease and certainly helped this group of patients. In 1993, my research group and I were honoured to have our work on the antiphospholipid syndrome recognized with the title 'Hughes' syndrome'.

Other advances

Many improvements in treatment have occurred in the second half of the twentieth century, these being the more conservative use of steroids, the use of immunosuppressive drugs, such as azathioprine and cyclophosphamide, and the more widespread and measured use of antimalarials.

At the same time, other advances in medicine have directly helped lupus sufferers. The better drugs now available to treat blood pressure, dialysis, transplantation, better sun-protection agents, and successful treatments for peptic ulcers and osteoporosis—to name but a few.

However, in terms of overall prognosis and outlook, it is probable that the twentieth-century's most lasting contribution has been better education and awareness about lupus—not only by patients, but also by doctors.

21 Research on lupus

Introduction

If you were in charge of a lupus research programme, where would you start? Perhaps by looking at some of the more obvious questions raised in clinical practice:

- Why the nine to one female predominance?
- Is there truly a genetic tendency?
- Why the aberrations in the immune system?
- How can we improve present medical treatment?
- Why do some patients have kidney disease, others thrombosis or skin rashes—and others not?

Research already demonstrates that there are considerable grounds for optimism in lupus. Although the disease was previously underfunded by many research-grant-giving bodies, there is at last a major or worldwide research effort in lupus. For example, areas of interest and research findings are now published in an international journal *Lupus*, which has a distinguished editorial board and attracts an enormous number of research papers.

Every two years, there is an international research meeting on lupus, the last three being in London, Jerusalem, and Cancun, Mexico. The next meeting will be in 2001, in Barcelona. Each meeting attracted nearly 1000 doctors and research workers. These meetings are models of scientific hard work and collaboration, bringing together clinicians, immunologists, clotting experts, obstetricians, and patient support groups. The large number of abstracts (written summaries of work) generated at these meetings, which are published in the journal *Lupus*, provide information on 'what's new in lupus' research for anyone interested. Work being undertaken is extensive but some of the main directions in research are summarized below.

Epidemiology

This is the study of the geography and national differences in lupus from country to country. From comparisons of the disease in different ethnic groups, we hope to gain insight into some of the environmental as well as genetic influences on the disease. Issues of the journal *Lupus* carry articles devoted to these topics in a series called 'Lupus around the world'.

Hormones

All the clinical evidence suggests that lupus is influenced by hormones. Certainly, the female hormone estrogen has a powerful effect on the immune response, and much work is now focused on hormones and hormone receptors (the sites in the body upon which hormones work) in patients with the disease. Lessons are being learnt from hormone studies in other diseases—such as in the management of breast cancer, where manipulation of hormone levels is already proving a useful form of treatment.

Today, hormones are not actively used in lupus because the side effects of the chemicals currently available are too many. However, the world of pharmacology is tenacious and future treatment may well come from this line of research.

Genetics

Each year, the tools for looking at genetic aspects of a disease become more precise. Twenty-five years ago, we were largely limited to blood groups. Now, DNA analysis makes genetic interpretation far more focused. Thus, intense research is now being studied on lupus patients and their families. As technology has advanced, the need for more careful clinical input into such studies has become more urgent. It is no longer acceptable to send out questionnaires asking if lupus exists in a family. The 'variations' of the clinical face of lupus range from migraine to recurrent miscarriages, atypical multiple sclerosis, schizophrenia, thyroid disease, multiple allergies, vein thrombosis, and rheumatism—to name but a few.

Genetic studies need to take these and other potentially lupus-related topics on board. Although the future discovery of a 'lupus gene' may not help cure the disease, it is possible that genetic factors will be found that affect disease expression and severity.

Immunology

The immune response is overactive in lupus. Obviously, this is so, but why? And what are the reasons behind this overactivity?

Conventional wisdom has it that there are two immunologically active cells: B-cells (the foot soldiers and producers of antibodies); and T-cells (the governing cells). In lupus, there is a failure of the 'suppressor' T-cells (the police force).

Anarchy prevails—the B-cells go 'wild' and overproduce antibody without an effective brake on their activity. Too much antibody 'clogs up' the system. Research groups worldwide are looking at this immunological mechanism found in lupus. For example, the thymus gland—an organ whose primary function is in regulating the immune system—is centrally involved in 'programming' certain immune cells. A few years ago, a group of patients were reported to have developed lupus some years after removal of the thymus gland. Some of these patients were in their fifties and sixties. The implication is that the normal thymus gland might have been performing a 'calming' regulatory role on the immune system.

Thrombosis

For my own research team, the discovery that some of the problems of lupus patients relate to thrombosis (blood clotting) has provided the focus of a huge research effort. One of the many antibodies produced in lupus—antiphospholipid antibody—is very strongly associated with thrombosis. This antibody appears to affect both the platelets and other clotting mechanisms, and has achieved importance well beyond the confines of lupus. What we described as the 'primary' anticardiolipin or antiphospholipid syndrome (APS) during the years 1983–5 has become recognized as an important and treatable clotting mechanism in strokes, heart attacks, thrombosis when taking the pill, and placental thrombosis (recurrent abortion)—to name but a few. The advantages to lupus patients and those with APS have been clear. For example, in our lupus pregnancy clinic, where some of the patients with antiphospholipid antibodies have had as many as eight to ten spontaneous miscarriages, the pregnancy success rate in the past fifteen years has risen from under 20% to over 70%!

Collaborative research studies

Increasingly, the emphasis is on collaboration. Within hospitals, such as ours at St Thomas', there are combined studies going on with different specialists such as immunologists, psychiatrists, nephrologists (kidney), and haematologists (blood). Internationally, the lupus world is small. The international journal, the international lupus meeting, the international antiphospholipid meeting, small meetings, such as the European lupus meeting, where lupus researchers touch base with colleagues in other disciplines, have each contributed to collaborative research links, over and above the more 'formal' societies of rheumatology, haematology, and so on.

Treatment

In every major clinical lupus unit in the world research goes on. There are no wonder drugs in sight—but then there never are until a 'new' advance is sprung on us.

The 'advances' most commonly come from the 'fine-tuning' of existing therapy—the move to lower dose steroids, low dose pulse cyclophosphomide regimes, combinations, etc. These seemingly small advances, taken together, have undoubtedly contributed significantly to the vastly improved prognosis of modern lupus.

22
Lupus around the world

Introduction

The world map of lupus has been redrawn completely during the past thirty-five years. In the 1960s, lupus was thought to be vanishingly rare in a number of countries, including Britain, most European countries, Africa, South America, and Australia, to name but a few. Indeed, the publication of series of more than 200 patients from any one clinic was largely confined to a few large centres, mainly in the United States. This situation has now totally reversed and there are large lupus clinics in almost every city in the world.

It is impossible to know whether the prevalence of lupus (the number of cases in a given population at any time) varies greatly, as these studies have been very difficult to carry out. The clinical impression, however, is that there are variations in the prevalence of this disease from country to country and continent to continent. In certain countries in the Far East, such as Malaysia, Singapore, and Indonesia, lupus has overtaken rheumatoid arthritis in its prevalence and, rheumatoid arthritis is now regarded as a less common disease. This is certainly true at St Thomas', London. The same may well be occurring in other countries, such as Jamaica, where lupus is a very common disease. In South America, the large cities have very large lupus clinics and, in all the Mediterranean countries where I have lectured lupus clinics are big and extremely busy. There are national lupus societies in almost every country, including China, Russia, the Far East, and most Middle Eastern countries.

In Africa, where lupus was once considered rare, it is now recognized that this was probably never the case. Large clinics exist in South Africa and I remember visiting a ward in Barragwanath Hospital, in one of the townships outside Johannesburg, and seeing large numbers of lupus patients. Possibly in some of these countries, other diagnoses for the joint pains, fever, and so on had been made prior to the recognition of the importance of lupus.

Is lupus increasing worldwide?

For the purist the answer must be 'we do not know'. It is certainly likely that the increase in the numbers of lupus patients is due to the increased recognition of milder cases, but I really cannot believe that physicians in the past were missing so many instances of this disease. I believe that there is a real increase in worldwide prevalence of lupus. There is no pattern from country to country, at the present time, to suggest an infectious etiology. For example, there are very few reports of clusters of lupus cases in small towns or villages. In addition, research has not yet thrown up a direct cause and effect relationship between the dwindling ozone layer, ultraviolet light exposure, and the possible rising prevalence of lupus, but doubtless this will become a focus of attention in the years to come. It is certainly true that there is a disparity between the number of cases of lupus diagnosed in greyer northern climes such as Scotland, for example, and sunny countries, such as Egypt and Greece, and whatever the cause of lupus, it must remain true that exposure to ultraviolet light is clearly an important precipitating factor.

Appendix: So you think you have lupus?

- Which specialist should you see?
- How can I influence my doctor?
- What do case studies show us?

Your doctor's view

So many patients with lupus seem to have had a long and fraught journey before a diagnosis is made and appropriate clinical treatment instituted. Lupus is one of the great mimics of all diseases and (to take the doctor's side) it is a disease that is very easily misdiagnosed. Until the last fifteen years or so it was thought to be rare. Putting oneself in the position of the average general practitioner, the likelihood of the number of new cases of lupus seen in a medical lifetime may well be small. That said, however, the same argument applies for dozens of rare diseases, and it is the job of the GP to be able to point the patient towards a specialist in that particular disease. Obviously, there are many patients who have the non-specific symptoms described in this book, who have either another disease, or no disease at all, and this is where the long medical training of doctors does come into play. We are lucky to have reasonably good screening tests for lupus; first, the antinuclear antibody (ANA test, see Chapter 4), which is generally positive in lupus (as well as in a number of other conditions) and, second, the anti-DNA antibody test which is more specific but sometimes negative in the milder forms of the disease (see Chapter 4).

If you think you or one of your family has lupus, by all means approach your GP, go through the normal medical channels, and ask to have a blood test for the disease. Also, ask to have a standard urine test for proteinuria if lupus is suspected by your doctor. Specialists who deal mostly in lupus in countries throughout the world are rheumatologists, dermatologists, and nephrologists (kidney specialists). Obviously, it matters little which specialist ends up treating you provided he or she knows about the disease, knows about its variability, and is prepared to take advice from colleagues. There has been an enormous growth worldwide in specialists dealing with lupus and this is paralleled by the rise in the number of doctors attending national and international research conferences on lupus.

Perhaps one of the most important trends has been the formation of 'teams' of doctors to run lupus clinics. For example, at the St Thomas' Hospital Lupus Unit, London, we have rheumatologists, nephrologists, ophthalmologists, psychiatrists, and obstetricians all taking part in our various weekly clinics.

Surely things must improve even further for the medical management of the lupus patient!

Appendix: Useful addresses

Many countries have their own national associations which do important work in raising awareness of the lupus disease. They also provide a network where patients, if they wish, can meet and discuss things with other patients and patient groups.

Some of the main addresses are as follows:

Australia
Lupus Association of NSW
PO Box 89
North Ryde 2113
New South Wales

Canada
Lupus Canada
P O Box 64034 5512-4 St NW
Calgary, AB T2K 6J1
Tel:/Fax: 403 274 5599
800-661-1468

Europe
European Lupus Erythematosus
Federation (ELEF)
St James House
Eastern Road
Romford
Essex RM1 3NH
Tel: 44 1708 73 12 51
Fax: 44 1708 73 12 52

Israel
Irgun Ha-Lupus 9e-Yisrael
c/o Margelit Nussinov/Miri
Rosenkovitch
10 Harav Nissim St
Raanana 43228
Tel: 972 4 71 40 27
Fax: 972 9 91 74 54

United Kingdom
Lupus UK
St James House
Eastern Road
Romford
Essex RM1 3NH
Tel: 44 1708 73 12 51
Fax: 44 1708 73 12 52

United States
Lupus Foundation of America Inc
1300 Piccard Drive, Suite 200
Rockville, MD 20850–4303
USA
Tel: (301) 670 9292
Fax: (301) 670 9486

Further reading

General

Isenberg, D. and Morrow, J. (1995). *Friendly fire*. Oxford University Press, Oxford. (160 pp.) (Autoimmune disease is explained)

Wallace, D. J. (1995). *The Lupus book*. Oxford University Press, Oxford.

Newsletter, books, fact sheets, and videos available from the Lupus UK Head Office: Lupus UK at St James House, Eastern Road, Romford, Essex RM1 3NH.

Aladjem, H. (1999). *The challenges of lupus*. Avery Publishing Group, New York.

Hughes, G. R. V. (1997). *Hughes' syndromes: a patient's guide to the antiphospholipid syndrome*. Lupus UK, Romford.

Scientific journal

Lupus—An International Journal. (Published every two months). Stockton Press, Basingstoke, UK.

Textbooks

Hughes, G. R. V. (1995). *Connective tissue diseases*, (4th edn). Blackwell Scientific, Oxford.

Lahita, R. G. (1999). *Systemic lupus erythematosus*, (3rd edn). Churchill Livingstone, Edinburgh. (1051 pp.)

Wallace, D. J. and Hahn, B. (1993). *Dubois' lupus erythematosus*, (4th edn). Lea & Febiger, Philadelphia. (955 pp.)

Glossary

ACTH Adreno-cortico-trophic-hormone. The natural hormone ('steroid') secreted in the body.

Adrenal gland A pair of glands situated above the kidney, responsible for making steroids.

Agoraphobia Fear of open spaces.

Albumin A protein, tested for in the urine. Increased amounts 'leak' into the urine when the kidney is inflamed.

Allergen A substance or chemical capable of causing an allergic reaction.

Alopecia Hair loss.

ANA (antinuclear antibody) The main screening test for lupus.

Anaemia A lack of the normal amount of red blood.

Antibodies Proteins produced by the body's immune system in defence against infection and other 'foreign' invasion.

Anticoagulant Drugs used to thin the blood (e.g. warfarin, heparin).

Atabrine Another name for mepacrine (an antimalarial drug).

Autoimmune disease A disease in which the immune system attacks elements of the patient's own body.

B-cell One of the groups of immune cells (lymphocytes).

Benign Generally used in defining lumps when they are not malignant.

Beta-blockers A group of drugs useful for damping down excessively fast heart rates and reducing high blood pressure.

Casein One of the proteins in cheese.

Chilblains A term used to describe cold blisters on the fingers, toes, or ears.

Cholesterol One of the body's circulating fat substances.

Claustrophobia Fear of confined spaces.

Cognition Awareness; ability to think methodically.

CRP (C-reactive protein) A blood protein. Raised levels are found in inflammation such as infections.

Cystitis Bladder inflammation.

Dermatomyositis Muscle inflammation (skin rashes may also occur, hence the 'dermato' part of the term).

Diuretics Pills which increase fluid excretion.

DNA The chemical in the nucleus which carries the genetic code.

Electroretinography A sensitive screening test for early abnormalities of the retina of the eye.

Endocarditis Inflammation of the inside wall of the heart (most commonly the heart valves).

Epilepsy Seizures due to abnormal 'electrical' discharges from the brain.

ESR (erythrocyte sedimentation rate) The blood test used as a 'barometer' of inflammation.

Etiology The cause of an illness.

Florid Gross or extreme.

Haemoglobin The protein molecule in red cells responsible for carrying oxygen around the body.

Herpes zoster See Shingles.

Hydrotherapy Physiotherapy in a pool.

Immunologist Doctor and/or scientist who studies the immune response.

ITP (idiopathic thrombocytopenic purpura) Low platelet count ('idiopathic' means that the cause is not yet determined).

Jaundice Yellowness of the skin due to the pigment bilirubin—can mean liver disease.

LE Lupus erythematosus.

Livedo reticularis A blotchy, purplish discoloration of blood vessels, usually on the wrists and knees.

Lymph glands Glands situated strategically around the body to protect against the spread of infection.

MCTD Mixed connective tissue disease.

ME Myalgic encephelopathy (disparagingly known as 'yuppie flu').

MRI (magnetic resonance imaging) The form of scan using magnetism rather than X-rays.

Nephritis Inflammation of the kidney.

Neuropathy Disease of the nerves.

Neuropsychiatric Involving normal and abnormal function of the brain.

Nivaquine One of the trade names for the antimalarial, chloroquine.

NSAIDs Non-steroidal anti-inflammatory drugs (standard anti-rheumatic drugs).

Nucleoproteins The complex proteins found in the nucleus of the cell.

Obstetrician Specialist dealing with pregnancy.

Opthalmoscope Instrument used to examine the eye.

Osteoporosis Fragile bone.

Pericarditis Inflammation of the delicate tissue membrane surrounding the heart.

Pericardium Membrane surrounding the heart.

Petit mal A form of epilepsy. Often takes the form of transitory 'absences'.

Physiotherapy Treatment by physical means.

Platelets The components of the blood responsible for clot formation.

Pleura The delicate tissue membrane surrounding the lungs.

Pleurisy Inflammation of the pleura, the delicate tissue membrane around the lungs.

Potassium One of the most important elements in the body's metabolism.

Proteinuria Presence of protein in the urine.

Psoriasis Chronic skin disorder—differs from lupus but is sometimes confused with skin lupus.

Psychosis Grossly abnormal, pathological behaviour pattern.

Puerperium The period of time after delivery of a baby.

Purpura Red spots under the skin—due to 'leaky' small blood vessels or to very low platelet counts.

Rhinitis Inflammation in the nose.

RNA (ribonucleic acid) Nucleic acids found in all living cells. They play an important part in protein synthesis.

Sclera The white of the eyes.

Schizophrenia Severely affected thought process. Characterized by auditory hallucinations ('voices').

SCLE Subacute cutaneous lupus erythematosus: an ultraviolet light-sensitive skin rash in lupus.

Scleritis Inflammation (and redness) in the white of the eye.

Septrin An antibiotic—often causes rashes in lupus patients.

Shingles A painful skin rash due to the virus, herpes zoster.

Sodium valproate A drug used in epilepsy.

Sputum Phlegm coughed up from the chest.

Steroids Chemicals manufactured by the adrenal glands. Now manufactured synthetically for medical use.

Streptococcal Infection with the bacterium, _Streptococcus_—can cause sore throats and (rarely) rheumatic fever.

Sulphonamides A group of antibiotics—now largely replaced by newer antibiotics.

Tartrazine A colouring used in foods which has been suggested can trigger lupus.

T-cell One of the groups of immune cells (lymphocytes).

Thalidomide A drug rarely used because of its disastrous side effects in pregnancy, but proving useful in some patients with severe skin lupus.

Thrombocytopenia Low platelet count.

Thrombosis Clotting of blood.

Tinnitus Ringing in the ears—may be associated with overuse of certain drugs such as aspirin.

Vasculitis Inflammation of the blood vessels.

The following terms are not defined in the Glossary but are explained in more detail in the chapters listed below:

ANA (antinuclear antibody) test Chapter 4.
Antiphospholipid syndrome (Hughes' syndrome) Chapter 15.
Anti-Ro/Anti-SSA Chapter 4.
Anti-Sm Chapter 4.
Azathioprine Chapter 5.
Behçet's disease Chapter 18.
Casts Chapter 3.
Chorea Chapter 15.
Complement (including C3 and C4) Chapter 3.
Cyclophosphamide Chapter 5.
Cyclosporin Chapter 5.
Discoid lupus Chapter 16.
ENA test Chapter 4.
Gammaglobulin Chapter 6.
Haemolytic anaemia Chapter 3.
Polyarteritis nodosa Chapter 18.
Prothrombin ratio Chapter 6.
Rheumatoid arthritis Chapter 18.
Scleroderma Chapter 18.
Sicca syndrome Chapter 17.
Sinusitis Chapter 18.
Sjögren's syndrome Chapter 17.
Still's disease Chapter 18.
Wegener's granulomatosis Chapter 18.

Index

Index

Index